Consanguinity Inbreeding and Autism:
An Anthropological Quest

Consanguinity Inbreeding and Autism:
An Anthropological Quest

Profulla C. Sarker
Nazir M Hossain

Copyright © 2024 by Profulla C. Sarker & Nazir M Hossain.

Library of Congress Control Number:		2024910934
ISBN:	Hardcover	979-8-3694-2276-2
	Softcover	979-8-3694-2275-5
	eBook	979-8-3694-2323-3

All rights reserved. No part of this book may be reproduced or transmitted in any form or by any means, electronic or mechanical, including photocopying, recording, or by any information storage and retrieval system, without permission in writing from the copyright owner.

Any people depicted in stock imagery provided by Getty Images are models, and such images are being used for illustrative purposes only.
Certain stock imagery © Getty Images.

Print information available on the last page.

Rev. date: 07/09/2024

To order additional copies of this book, contact:
Xlibris
844-714-8691
www.Xlibris.com
Orders@Xlibris.com
803078

CONTENTS

Dedication xi
Preface xiii
Acknowledgments xv

Chapter 1 Introduction 1

Historical Background 1
Religious Views of Marriage 2
Views of Marriage in Hinduism 3
Views of Marriage in Islam 4
Views of Marriage in Christianity 6
Views of Marriage in Buddhism 6
Practice of Consanguineous Marriage 7
Consanguinity and Autism 8
Global Scenario of Consanguinity 11
Religious Views on Consanguineous Mariage 13
Discourse of Consanguinity on Autism 15
Concluding Remarks 15

Chapter 2 Methods and Techniques Applied to Conduct Research 22

Introduction 22
Theoretical Framework 22
Objectives of the Study 25
Research Questions 26
Expected Results 26
Sampling Procedure 27
Research Design 27
Methods of Data Collection 29
Research Report 30
Outlines of Research Report 31
Concluding Remarks 31

Chapter 3   Consanguineous Marriages in Cross-Cultural Perspective 34

Introduction 34
Consanguineous Marriage in Regionality 35
Consanguinity in Cross-Cultural Perspective 36
Consanguineous Marriages in Bangladesh 40
Types of Consanguineous Marriage 42
Symbols of Kinship Relations 43
Reasons for Consanguineous Marriage 44
Concluding Remarks 46

Chapter 4   Sociodemographic Profile of the Parents and the Autistic Children 49

Introduction 49
Age Structure of Parents 50
Level of Education of Parents 51
Occupation Structure of Parents 52
Family Types of Autistic Children 53
Authority Structure of Family 54
Gender-Specific Age of Autistic Children 56
Categories of Autism Spectrum Disorders 57
Concluding Remarks 58

Chapter 5   Signs and Symptoms of Autism Spectrum Disorders (ASD) 60

Introduction 60
Evidence of Autism Spectrum Disorders 61
Sing and Symtoms of ASD 61
Causes of Autism Spectrum Disorders 65
Characteristics of Autism Spectrum Disorders 66
Restricted Interests and Repetitive Behavior 67
Concluding Remarks 67

Chapter 6   Consanguinity, Gene Mutation, and Inbreeding Their Impact on ASD 70

Introduction 70

Consanguinity and Genetic Risk 71
Consanguinity 72
Inbreeding 73
Gene Mutation through Consanguinity 74
Impact on Consanguinity 77
Concluding Remarks 78

Chapter 7   Perceptions, Beliefs, and Myths about Autism Spectrum Disorder 81

Introduction 81
Parents' Perception of ASD 82
Beliefs in the Etiology of ASD 83
Myths and Facts about Autism 84
Concluding Remarks 95

Chapter 8   Diagnosis, Treatment, and Knowledge of Parents about Treatment 99

Introduction 99
Early Signs and Symptoms 100
Diagnosis of Autistic Children 101
Developmental Screening 102
Comprehensive Diagnostic Evaluation 102
Diagnostic Features of ASD 103
Diagnostic Tools 103
Diagnostic Guideline 104
Treatment Processes 105
Treatment Options 106
Management of Health 107
Future Planning 107
Challenges to High-Functioning Autism 108
Strengths in High-Functioning Autism 109
Parents' Knowledge of Treatment 109
Treatment Options in the Research Area 110
Parents' Access to Treatments 111
Challenges to Get Treatment 112
Concluding Remarks 112

Chapter 9 Challenges for Parents and Families in Raising Autistic Children 116

Introduction 116
Challenges for Parents Families 117
Concluding Remarks 126

Chapter 10 Problems Faced by Autistic Children at the Family Level 131

Introduction 131
Autism and Related Problems 132
Felt Unpleasant Emotion 132
Language Communication 133
Regulatory and Sensory-Motor 133
Self-Stimulatory Behaviors 133
Problems at the Family Level 134
Anxiety of the Autistic Children 137
Challenges to Autistic Children 137
Daily Life Challenges 139
Concluding Remarks 142

Chapter 11 Initiatives of GOs, NGOs, and POs about Autism Spectrum Disorders 145

Introduction 145
Action Plan against Autism 146
Programs for Autism 147
Services to the Autistic Children 148
Acts Mitigating Autism 148
Bangladesh in Global Setting 149
Observance of National Autism Day 151
National Advisory Committee 151
National Policy on Autism 152
Autism School and Therapy Center 153
Concluding Remarks 154

**Chapter 12 Life Cycle-Focused ASD Prevention and
               Rehabilitation Strategy** 156

Introduction 156
Stages of the Human Life Cycle 157
Life Cycle-Focused Prevention Strategy 158
Strategy before Conception 159
Rehabilitation Strategies 164
Concluding Remarks 172

**Chapter 13 Counseling against Consanguinity for Inbred
               Community** 182

Introduction 182
Concept of Genetic Counseling 183
Genetic Counseling in Bangladesh 184
Process of Genetic Counselling 185
Role of Genetic Counselor 187
Tips in Counseling against Consanguinity 188
Concluding Remarks 189

**Chapter 14 Training for Parents of Children with Autism
               Spectrum Disorder** 194

Introduction 194
Discrete Trial Training for the Parents 195
Significance of Training for the Parents 196
Methods of Training for the Parents 198
Role of Parent in Psychosocial Functioning 205
Concluding Remarks 206

**Chapter 15 Conclusions and Policy Implications on Autism
               Spectrum Disorders** 216

Introduction 216
Policies for Bangladesh 218
Concluding Remarks 224
Glossary 227
Index 243
About the Authors 249

Dedication

"To those parents who dedicated their entire lives to the happiness of their special child."

Preface

The research interest in autistic disorders is increasing among scholars in the discipline of genetics, medical science, and social science across the world, especially where consanguineous marriages are preferred. Research in consanguinity is also increasing in the Arab world, particularly in Egypt and Saudi Arabia, as evidenced in the last few years. Studies revealed that the research on autism in Arab countries is still in its infancy and needs organizational efforts to be fruitful because consanguineous marriages are widely practiced over there. On the other hand, consanguineous marriages are famous in some communities in South Asian countries, including Bangladesh; unfortunately, nobody has done any intensive research absolutely on consanguinity and its effects on autism spectrum disorder (ASD).

The studies also revealed that consanguinity enables the identification of genetic risk. The recent interest and rapid expansion in genetic research made possible by molecular analysis techniques that date from the mid-1980s, and now also by advanced methods of next-generation genomic sequencing, continues to open new possibilities for preventing the births of children with severe genetic conditions. Alongside this technical development, there has been a parallel expansion in public and academic engagements with genetic research and its social and ethical implications. The understanding of genetic risk is being incorporated into the health policies of many countries throughout the world to avoid consanguineous marriages and prevent autism.

So far, the knowledge of the authors goes that there has not been any significant research on consanguinity, inbreeding, and the probability of autism in inbred communities. It is clear from the literature review and the findings of this research that previous researchers have done most of the research on consanguinity and its impact on reproductive health. They partially included autism as one of the segments of reproductive health, which is relevant to the existing study. It has been found in different studies that in developing countries and specifically in the Arab world along with South Asian Countries, the field of child psychiatry is relatively new. Autism spectrum spectrum spectrum spectrum spectrum spectrum Spectrum Disorder (ASD) became a subject of interest in these regions only during the late 1990s. Tremendous effort is needed to raise policymakers' awareness of the need for the implementation of services and research plans aimed at bridging the gap between the needs and services provided for autism. Under the circumstances, this volume examines to what extent the consanguinity in terms of cross-cousin and parallel-cousin marriages affects autism in the inbred community of Bangladesh.

The findings of this research will contribute to the knowledge of scientists, academics, researchers, clinicians, students, and a wide range of fields, including administrators, planners, policymakers, and practitioners, to prevent autism by providing counseling to people to avoid consanguineous marriages and, at the same time, to educate the parents of autistic children on how to take care of their children, involving the cooperation and supports of the GOs, NGOs, INGOs, and VOs to make the autistic children as productive members of the society to lead an everyday life with the fulfillment of basic needs and civic facilities like other members.

Profulla C. Sarker and Nazir M Hossain

Acknowledgments

This volume, entitled *Consanguinity, Inbreeding, and Autism: An Anthropological Quest*, is based on the report of the research project on "Consanguinity and Its Impact on the Probability of Autism in an Inbred Community of Bangladesh" conducted by the authors in Dhaka Metropolitan City in the year 2020–2021. Many people were involved in different capacities with this research project. They were field investigators, research associates, and informants. In addition, the Social Science Research Council and special education schools were involved in organizational capacity to make the research project successful. The authors are indebted to the Social Science Research Council for providing financial support in conducting this research project and, at the same time, are grateful to the different special education school authorities for allowing them to collect data about autistic children and their parents.

Special thanks and gratitude are due to the parents of the autistic children for providing personal as well as sensitive information. The researchers are also thankful to the key informants and members of the FGD groups for their active participation, support, and cooperation in providing valuable information on consanguinity and its effects on autism. The researchers appreciated the contribution of Dr. Md. Shafiqur Rahman, who provided valuable comments and suggestions to improve the quality of the research report. As an expert on public health, the researchers is indebted to him for editing this volume.

The researchers sincerely thank Najnin Sultana, Sheuli Roy Ritu, Khadija Binte Habib, and Habibur Rahman for their thorough job and responsibility for data collection, especially during the pandemic. Thanks are also due to research associate Shaidul Islam for data editing and data processing and Ahmed Abdullah for technical support in preparing graphs for quantitative data analysis. The researcher also expresses his sincere thanks to Md. Zakir Hossain for his support when computing the research report; otherwise, completing the research project would not have been possible.

The authors of this volume are indebted to the authority of Sheikh Hasina University of Science and Technology, especially the chairman, Board of Trustees, Dr. HMB Iqbal, for permitting them to conduct this research and allowing to publish this research report as a book in the aegis of the Center for Research, Knowledge Management, and Human Resource Development. The researchers would like to sincerely thank the Social Science Research Council staff under the Ministry of Planning, the People's Republic of the Government of Bangladesh, for continuous communication and cooperation, which helped the research progress. Finally, the researchers could complete the research project in the scheduled time and publish this report as a book.

Finally, the authors thank their family members for encouraging them to participate in this research project and for preparing this manuscript for publication as a book.

Profulla C. Sarker and Nazir M Hossain

Chapter 1

INTRODUCTION

Historical Background

The most and the best available evidence suggests that marriage is about 4,350 years of biosocial institution. For thousands of years, most anthropologists believed that families consisted of loosely organized groups of as many as thirty people, with several male leaders and multiple women shared by them and their children. As the hunter-gatherers settled into agrarian civilizations, society needed more stable socioeconomic arrangements by institutionalizing marriage in human societies. The first recorded evidence of marriage ceremonies uniting a woman and a man dated from about 2350 BC in Mesopotamia. Over the next several hundred years, marriage became a widespread institution the ancient Hebrews, Greeks, and Romans embraced. Nevertheless, marriage had little to do with love or religion among the spouses; instead, it encouraged the production of legitimate offspring to increase the family members' biological and social satisfaction (Prayson 2016).

The primary purpose of marriage was to bind women and men together, thus guaranteeing that a man's children were his biological heirs. It is believed that a woman became a man's property through marriage. In the betrothal ceremony of ancient Greece, a father would hand over his daughter with these words: "I pledge my daughter for producing legitimate offspring." Studies have found that men were free to take several wives by marriage among the ancient Hebrews. Greek and Roman men were free to satisfy their sexual urges with concubines, prostitutes, and even teenage male lovers. At the same time, their wives were required to stay home and tend to household activities, as well as the care of children and dependence. If wives failed to produce offspring, especially male heirs, their husbands could give them back to their natal residence and marry again with someone else. As the Roman Catholic Church became a powerful institution in Europe, the blessings of a priest became a necessary step for a marriage to be legally recognized. By the eighteenth century, marriage was widely accepted in the Catholic church as a sacrament or a ceremony to bestow God's grace. At the Council of Trent in 1563, the sacramental nature of marriage was written into canon law.

Church blessings did improve the quality of life and well-being of the wives. Men were taught to show tremendous respect for their wives and forbidden from divorcing them. Christian doctrine declared that "the twain shall be one flesh," giving husband and wife exclusive access to each other's body, mind, and soul. This put new pressure on the mindset of the men to remain sexually faithful to their existing wives. However, the church still held that men were the heads of families, and the authority of the families was in the hands of the husbands; that is, a patriarchal family system emerged.

Different studies have found the keen interest behind consanguineous marriage to keep wealth and power within the family, especially in a kinship network system. The Pharaohs often married their sister or half-sister, and after a handful of generations, the offspring were mentally and physically unfitted to rule. Another historical example is the royal houses of Europe, where royal families often married each other because tradition did not allow them to marry people of non-royal class or outside of kinship ties. As a result, it affected the mental retardation and physical deformation of their offspring, and ultimately, they became unfit to rule.

Religious Views of Marriage

Marriage is a universal practice in South Asia among people of different religions: Hinduism, Islam, Christianity, and Buddhism. Marriage is solemnized in various groups based on religious rites and ceremonies. Marriage is also solemnized based on either sacramental or contractual or both. It should be noted that the Hindu and the Buddha marriage in Bangladesh is primarily sacramental, but registration is secondary. On the other hand, Muslim and Christian marriage is contractual. Every religion encourages marriage to increase followers by producing offspring as a part of their religious duty. The meaning of marriage may differ from the perspective of cultural variations and different segments of the population of the same religion. In ancient times, for example, marriage meant a condition in which a woman was given to a man almost as property. In the diachronic process of change in human history, marriage becomes a permanent institution that, once entered, cannot be dissolved except by the death of one of the spouses. In addition, marriage may be declined legally in the modern world for specific legitimate reasons.

The meaning of marriage can be looked at from a legal perspective. Legally, marriage is a binding contract between the two parties that combines their possessions, income, and lives. The state recognizes marriage, and the dissolving of the contract can only happen through the legal process of divorce. However, for most people, marriage has meaning beyond the legal sense. Marriage is also an agreement between the man and woman. Husband and wife take certain vows to love one another, to cherish one another, and to stay together through sickness and health, for better and for worse. In most cases, this agreement includes sexual faithfulness and a promise that each person will do what they can to make the other one happy. For some people, this agreement between man and woman takes the form of a covenant between them not only as a couple but also the will of God as well. Under these circumstances, many marriages are performed through rites and ceremonies based on the prescription of the respective religion.

Views of Marriage in Hinduism

Marriage is a universal practice among Hindus because a man is expected to go through the various stages of his life, performing the duties attached to each stage, and marriage is one of the duties. The Hindus are expected to pursue four goals in their life, viz., *dharma* (religious duty), *artha* (wealth), *Kama* (sex desire), and moksha (salvation, i.e., ultimate spiritual release). Keeping with these goals, the human life cycle is divided into four ashrams (stages): brahmacharya, *grihastha, vanaprastha,* and *sanyas* (Sindh 1974,

p. 140). A man enters the second stage, i.e., grihasthya, by getting married. So, marriage is universal and a compulsory duty in Hindu society. It is a religious duty ascribed to all people alike. In the life of a Hindu, marriage is an important landmark because it is one of the ten *sanskaras* (compulsory rites ascribed by sastras from religion).

The aims of a Hindu marriage are dharma (religion), Praja (progeny), and ratio (pleasure). When a woman gets married and becomes a householder, her aspects *of dharma are* the highest aim of marriage. Though sex is one of the functions of marriage, it is given third place, indicating thereby that it is the least desirable aim of marriage. For women, marriage is essential because, though a man goes through several sacraments throughout his life, marriage is the only sacrament for a woman that she is allowed (Bhende and Kanitkar 1982, p. 92). On the other hand, procreation is the second aim of marriage, and the highest objective is to bring forth a son. In the literature of Manusamhita and Mahabharata, a derivation of the word Putra (son) is who saves the father from going to *narak* or *put* (hell). On the other hand, a daughter is desired for *kanyadan* (offering a daughter to the groom). The place of children (both son and daughter) in the family is so elevated that the duty of procreation is for the family's interest, although it is not said to be the highest aim of marriage. Under the circumstances, Hindu thinkers regard marriage in the ideal sense as not so much for sex or for progeny but for obtaining a partner for the fulfillment of one's religious duty (Kapadia 1966, p. 67).

Views of Marriage in Islam

Marriage is a legal arrangement for Muslims, although it is imbued with religious overtones (Jacobson 1976, p. 182). Marriage is also considered a *sunna* (practices and precepts of the Prophet); therefore, it is regulated as an obligation that must be fulfilled. The objectives of marriage in Islam are not only to ensure the continuity of the lineage but also to increase the number of followers of Islam. In *sharia* (Islamic law), it is said that "when a servant of Allah marries, he perfects half of his religion" (Abul et al. 1924, p. 12). Islamic texts are also evident on the point that the primary objective of marriage is the satisfaction of sexual urge, which is achieved through sexual intercourse between husband and wife. Islam does not permit premarital, extramarital, or postmarital coitus of divorced and

Introduction

widowed women, which is considered as *guna* (sin) in the Islamic sense of the term. Postmarital sex refers to the coital activity of divorced, separated, and widowed women without marital ties. However, postmarital sex is less a social controversy than premarital and extramarital relations. Studies revealed that extramarital ties are more common among those who have experienced premarital coitus than those who have not. The Muslims look down upon unmarried persons because marriage is *mashhur* (very essential) to a Muslim for the procreation of sons and daughters, who thereby renews and extends his own life through them.

From the above analysis, marriage is essential for the Hindus and the Muslims as well in the context of religiosity. According to Hindu philosophy, marriage is a *sanskara* (reform), and as such, it is a sacrament and religious bond between husband and wife. At the same time, among Muslims, it provides a legal union that safeguards society from moral and social degradation. Ideally, it aims not only at the individual's biological, emotional, social, and spiritual fulfillment and development through union with a person of the opposite sex but also contributes to the family's development, fulfillment, and welfare (Kapur 1973, p. 6). According to traditional views of Hinduism, marriage is a social as well as religious duty toward the family and the community, and there is little idea of individual interest, while among the Muslims, the objective of marriage is to ensure the continuity of the lineage and to increase the number of followers of Islam.

In a village study of Bangladesh, it has been observed that apart from the ideal traditional view about marriage, people were giving importance to marriage for the fulfillment of biosocial as well as personal needs and happiness, that is, to satisfy the sexual urge and procreation of children along with the fulfillment of one's religious and social duties. Marriage is the only way to meet sexual desire, and any other sexual activity is considered a sin in the context of the religiosity of both religious groups. It is also believed that the procreation of offspring is the urging of parents, and they want to remain alive in the memory of their *santan-santati* (progeny). Procreation outside the marriage bond is uncommon in Bangladesh, except for the adoption among Hindus, Buddhists, and Christians (Maloney et al. 1981, p. 76).

Views of Marriage in Christianity

Most Christian denominations view marriage as a permanent and lifelong commitment between men and women. In Christianity, marriage is also considered a holy sacrament and a reflection of the relationship between Jesus Christ and the church. The views on marriage among the different sects of Christians are different. In Roman Catholic teachings, marriage expresses the purpose of man and woman. It is the basis for procreation and the symbolic expression of the union of Christ and the Catholic church. It also provides mutual support to the married couple and includes legitimacy for sexual relations between them. Traditionally, marriage is considered a contract between a man and a woman, consummated and respected, where each takes control of the other's body, and sexual congress is expected and welcomed. On the other hand, in Eastern Orthodox teachings, marriage is also considered a sacrament. Additionally, it is viewed as an ordination. This concept of ordination is deemed to be martyrdom, in which each spouse symbolically dies for the sake of the other and, in so doing, confirms and sanctifies the relationship. In Protestant denominations, marriage may vary in their doctrines but have some fundamental customs and beliefs in common. Most Protestant denominations view marriage as a union of a man and a woman, ordained by God, with the primary purpose being the celebration of God's love for the world. Marriage is also the vehicle for raising children and providing mutual help and support to each other (Sarker 2017).

Liberal theological Christians, in keeping with the overall view of individualism and personal interpretation, have taken a much more encompassing view of marriage. With a broader acceptance of humanity's infinite variety and acceptance that theological and philosophical tenets change as humanity progresses, the definitions of marriage are now evolving to include same-sex marriage, especially in the West.

Views of Marriage in Buddhism

Buddhism never had a religious statement on marriage, about holiness, either holy or unholy. Buddhism does not regard marriage as a sacrament that is ordained in heaven. However, it considers secular affairs. Buddhism allows everyone the freedom to decide all the issues about marriage. This does not mean that Buddhism is against marriage. Nobody in this world would say that marriage is wrong, and no religion is against marriage. Marriage is a personal and social obligation; it is not compulsory. Buddhist theologians have never defined what a proper marriage between lay Buddhists entails and generally do not preside over marriage ceremonies.

Buddhists are expected to follow the civil laws regarding marriage, which are laid out according to the rules and regulations of their respective government where they live. While the ceremony is civil, many Buddhists obtain blessings from monks (priests) at the local temple after the marriage is completed; however, religion does not require it. As per the Tibetan Buddhist encyclopedia, one should pay attention to the advice given by the Enlightened Teacher if one wants to lead a happy married life. In His discourses, the Buddha gave various advice for married couples and those contemplating marriage. The Buddha has said, "If a man can find a suitable and understanding wife and a woman can find a suitable and understanding husband, both are fortunate indeed," as a result, marriage is an ideal relationship between the husband and the wife to reproduce legitimate children.

Practice of Consanguineous Marriage

The practice of consanguineous marriage was common in earlier times, and it continues to be expected in some societies today, though, in some jurisdictions, such marriages are prohibited. Worldwide, more than 10 percent of marriages are between first and second cousins. Cousin marriage is an essential topic in medical science, anthropology, sociology, social work, genetics, and alliance theory of any allied disciplines (Ottenheimer 1996). In some cultures, cousin marriages are already considered ideal and are actively encouraged and expected; in others, they are seen as incestuous and are subject to social stigma and taboo. Cousin marriage was historically practiced by many indigenous cultures, such as Australia, New Zealand, North America, South America, and Polynesia (Dousset 2018).

In some jurisdictions, cousin marriage is legally prohibited in many East and West countries. For example, Australia, European countries, China, Taiwan, Thailand, some East Asian countries, South Korea, the Philippines, and twenty-four states out of the fifty states of North America (Paul and

Spencer 2008). In addition, cousin marriage is restricted among the Hindus in Bangladesh, North India, and so on. The laws of many jurisdictions set the degree of consanguinity restriction. Studies revealed that the children of first-cousin marriages have an increased risk of autosomal recessive genetic disorders, and this risk is higher in populations that are already highly ethnically similar. Children of more distantly related cousins have less risk of these disorders, though still higher than the average population (Hamamy 2012; White and Roberson-Nay 2009). It has already been identified in genetic research that to prevent autism, consanguineous marriage needs to be restricted.

Consanguinity and Autism

Recently, there has been increased interest in research on autism and the problems of autistic children across the world. However, it is found that autism is not a contagious disease. Since it is not contagious, there must be other forces that somehow create or pass on the autistic symptoms. The DNA reports show that deviations in the genetic code due to ancient inbreeding can follow a human line for generations. Studies indicate that inbreeding eventually produces autistic symptoms (Prayson 2016). Different studies have found that inbreeding was widespread until a few hundred years ago, and it continues today, but to a lesser degree.

After millions of inbreeds, the world population has become so numerous that it is globally sharing ancestors, producing genetic abnormalities (ibid). On the other hand, autism may be the result of the widespread inbreeding of ancient generations. Under the circumstances, the people are all touched by autism to one degree or another through common ancestors across the East and the West. Leavitt (2003) argued that consanguineous marriage does not produce congenital disabilities, but it increases the chances of inheriting a bad DNA fit, which results in congenital disabilities. The core features of autism were first described in Kanner's (1943) remarkable description of eleven children who showed a cluster of social, communicative, and behavioral features unique from other diagnostic entities such as mental retardation and childhood schizophrenia. The earliest autism diagnosis indicates that from the early 1943s until the 1960s, Kanner's premise, although incorrect, was that autism is caused by child neglect, withdrawal of affection, and, in general, poor parenting (Kanner 1943).

Introduction

In the 1970s, researchers determined that autism is not the result of emotional abuse; instead, it occurs due to gene mutation in consanguinity or consanguineous relationships through inbreeding. Under the circumstances, all human societies, either primitive or geographically isolated, prohibit the mating of first-degree relatives. Marriage between relatives less closely than siblings or parents and offspring is necessarily outlawed, but the dividing line between legal and illegal is hazy and varies from country to country. It should be noted that for about one-half of the total population of the United States of America, consanguineous marriage is prohibited by law (Maheswari and Wadhw 2016). Consanguineous marriage was also legally prohibited by the Chinese government in 1981. On the other hand, consanguineous marriage in South India is legal (ibid). It has been reported that in Bangalore and Mysore, two major cities of Karnataka state of south India, about 21 percent of marriages among the Hindus were consanguineous (Mehndirtta et al. 2007). Different studies have found that the detrimental health effects associated with consanguinity are caused by the expression of recessive genes inherited from common ancestors.

In Arab Muslim communities, first-cousin unions between a man and his father's brother's daughter are preferred. However, in the population of Dravidian Hindus of South India, the marriage of a boy with his mother's brother's daughter is opposed; instead, father's brother's daughter marriages are encouraged. This patrilineal cousin marriage is found in the patriarchal social system to keep their property within the family and strengthen kinship ties. On the other hand, uncle-niece unions but not aunt-nephews are permitted in Judaism. Studies indicate that consanguineous marriages are strongly favored in human populations in many societies worldwide. The highest consanguineous marriages, for example, 20 to over 50 percent, are reported in North Africa and Asia. Usually, consanguinity is associated with low socioeconomic status, illiteracy, and rural background (Grant and Bittles 1967; Bittles 2001). The main reasons for these marriages are stronger family ties, the integrity of estates, and the like. However, the current debate in medical sciences is on the health implications of these consanguineous marriages. Recently, Nalini et al. (2008) reported that consanguinity has a 46.4 percent role in causing dysferlinopathy in 28 patients. Further, Bindu et al. (2006) reported in their research that consanguinity is about 61.5 percent of the etiological factor for Hallervorden-Spatz syndrome (HSS). Reports from India and the West proved beyond doubt that consanguinity plays a significant role in mental health problems. All these disorders play a significant role in the world economy and productivity and become a massive burden on the medical fraternity. Despite medical advancements, an increase in literacy rate, and the expansion of urbanization, these family-linked traditions still need to be broken. In recent times, the situation appears better in urban areas. In a population with a high degree of inbreeding, formulating a public health program with a multi-approach strategy, including education about the anticipated genetic consequences, prenatal diagnosis, neonatal screening, and genetic counseling, is necessary.

Studies revealed that consanguineous marriages are major risk factors for bipolar disorders. This marriage system has been reported as an essential factor in the appearance of autosomal recessive diseases and congenital anomalies, including hydrocephalus, postaxial hand polydactyl and bilateral cleft lip cleft palate, bipolar disorders, depression, dysferlinopathy, reproductive disorders, sterility, infant mortality, child deaths, spontaneous abortions, and stillbirths, etc. Also, reports are indicating a positive association between consanguinity and Down syndrome, as well as a ventricular septal defect (VSD), atrial septal defect (ASD), atrioventricular septal defect (AVSD), pulmonary stenosis (PS), and pulmonary atresia (PA). The risk for congenital disabilities in the offspring of first-cousin mating has been increased to 5–8 percent compared to 2–3 percent in non-consanguineous marriages (Magnus et al. 1985). However, despite these health problems of the offspring health problems, the first cousin unions are culturally preferred in many societies. The reason is the ease of marriage decision-making when the potential spouse is well-known to each other and considered to be part of the extended family. These marriages also tend to reinforce social and kinship bonds from one generation to another next generation. The offspring of consanguineous unions are at increased risk for congenital disabilities, with the figure quoted for first-cousin unions' third-degree relatives of 1.7 to 2.8 percent (ibid). This is primarily due to autosomal recessive mutations inherited from a common ancestor but also includes disorders of putative multifactorial and complex inheritance, such as congenital heart defects (Stoltenberg et al. 1997; Yunis et al. 2006). Newborns are also more likely to have decreased birth weight (Mumtaz et al. 2007) and present with apnea of prematurity (Tamim et al. 2003) than newborns whose parents are not consanguineous.

Consanguineous pregnancies are also at a higher risk for adverse outcomes, such as miscarriages, stillbirths, neonatal and infant morbidity, and mortality (Bundey et al., 1990; Hussain, 1998). Although primary care practitioners are expected to collect information about family history, including consanguineous marriages, their perception of this role and any beliefs, barriers, or factors influencing the practice of consanguineous marriages are unknown. Although marriages in North America, most European countries, and Australia are not typically consanguineous, populations within these countries have higher consanguinity rates. This is due to migration from areas such as Africa, the Middle East, and South and Southeast Asia, where the rate of consanguinity is between 20 to 50 percent, especially among Muslims (Bennet et al. 2002). About 85 percent of the total population of Bangladesh is Muslim, and consanguineous marriage is allowed among them, but it does not mean that all marriages are consanguineous. Sociocultural, quasi-economic, and political factors are associated with consanguineous marriage among the Muslims of Bangladesh.

Global Scenario of Consanguinity

Consanguinity is a genetic concept that influences the probabilities of specific combinations of characteristics, called genotypes. The likelihood that two consanguineous individuals will share the same traits depends upon the mode of inheritance, either dominant or recessive, and the degree of penetrance or expressivity of the causative gene. Different studies have found that the higher rate of autism is more common in the offspring of consanguineous unions. While consanguineous marriages of various degrees have been practiced, all societies have incest taboos prohibiting marriage or sexual relations between certain kin.

People are all connected to life across the globe irrespective of geo-social boundaries, religious affiliations, and ethnicity. Every choice they make and every belief they hold influences the whole of life. Different studies have revealed that people live with the consequences of their choices. As part of biological health, this unique truth has physical expressions in honor, loyalty, family, and group bonds. This forms the basis of marriage, one of the most vital and powerful human relationships. The human population has seen modern civilization and is still within family boundaries. One of the most familial social bonds occurs through consanguineous marriages worldwide.

Consanguineous marriage is a marriage between closely related individuals. Though it may involve incest, it implies more than the sexual nature of incest. In a clinical sense, marriage between two family members who are second cousins or closer qualifies as consanguineous marriage. This is based on the gene copies their offspring may receive (Heidari et al. 2014). Though these unions are still prevalent in some communities across the greater Middle East region, many other populations have significantly declined intra-family marriages (Obeidat 2010). Globally, 8.5 percent of children have consanguineous parents, and 20 percent of the human population live in communities practicing endogamy (Akrami et al., 2009). Theories on the development of consanguineous marriage as a taboo can be supported as being both a social and a biological development because marriage is a biosocial network relationship between the husbands and wives irrespective of religion, ethnicity, class, sect, and geographical boundaries across the East and the West.

Consanguinity is a deeply rooted biosocial trend among one-fifth of the population worldwide, primarily residing in the Middle East, West Asia, some parts of South Asia, and North Africa (Hamamy 2012), which is discussed elsewhere in this chapter. The prevalence of consanguinity and rates of first-cousin marriage, either cross-cousin or parallel-cousin marriages, may vary widely within and between populations and communities, depending on ethnicity, religion, and culture regarding traditional customs, beliefs, values, and geography. Consanguineous marriages are also practiced among emigrant communities from highly consanguineous countries and regions, such as Afghanistan, Bangladesh, India, Iran, Iraq, Pakistan, Turkey, North Africa, and Lebanon, now resident in Europe, Canada, North America, Australia, and New Zealand (Schulpen et al. 2006). A world map is enclosed here in Figure 1 to give a clear idea of the percentage of consanguineous marriages from a global perspective. One billion people worldwide are estimated to live in communities that prefer consanguineous marriage (Bittles and Black 2010; Modell and Darr 2002). Consanguineous marriage is traditionally respected in most communities of North Africa, the Middle East, and West Asia, where intra-familial unions collectively account for 20 to more than 50 percent of all marriages (Tadmouri et al. 2009).

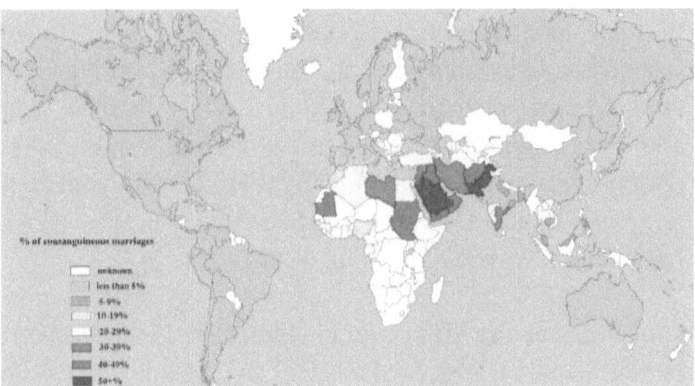

Fig. 1: Practice of Consanguineous Marriages across the World (Bittles 2011; Hamamy et al. 2011; Tadmouri et al. 2009)

Religious Views on Consanguineous Mariage

There is wide diversity in the views of the different religions toward consanguineous marriage. In general, consanguineous marriage is permitted within Judaism, in some segments of Christianity, Islam, Dravidian Hinduism, and Buddhism. However, the prevalence of specific types of consanguineous marriage is allowed in different religions under circumstances that vary from time to time. The following religions have different views toward consanguineous marriages.

- **Consanguineous Marriage in Islam:** In Islam, both first-cousin and double first-cousin marriages are allowed, whereas uncle-niece marriages are prohibited. The Quran contains no guidelines that encourage such marriages; even in one of the Hadith of Prophet Muhammad, cousin marriages are discouraged. However, he married his daughter Fatima to Ali, his paternal cousin (Hussain 1999). Thus, among this religious group, cousin marriages indicate following the path of the Prophet (Bittles, 2002). Studies revealed that cross-cousin and parallel-cousin marriage are widely practiced among Muslims throughout the world.

- **Consanguineous Marriage in Hinduism:** Hindus have a non-uniform attitude toward consanguinity. The Aryan Hindus of northern India prohibit it from approximately seven generations on the male side and five generations on the female side (Kapadia 1958). In contrast, Dravidian Hindus of south India favor consanguineous marriages between first cousins in Andhra Pradesh, Karnataka, and Tamil Nadu. In addition, niece marriages are also preferred (Bittles 2001). On the other hand, the Hindus of Bangladesh do not allow consanguineous marriage like the Aryan Hindus of northern India, and it is strictly prohibited.

- **Consanguineous Marriage in Buddhism:** Buddhism originated in North India in the third century BC, and the Prince Buddha is reputed to have married his first cousin. Perhaps for this reason, there is no overall proscription of consanguineous marriage within the Buddhist tradition. Instances of cross-cousin marriages in Pali literature are found only in the post-canonical stratum. They are unsupported or, in some cases, contradicted by non-Pali versions of the same stories. They reflect, therefore, the kinship practices of early Ceylon, not North India. Eighteen cases of cross-cousin marriage among Ceylonese kings are almost equally divided between the patrilateral (father's sister's daughter) and matrilateral (mother's brother's daughter) varieties, showing that the rule was bilateral. Ceylon's kings entered cross-cousin and parallel-cousin marriages to ensure the purity of descent and the internal harmony of the large, essentially endogamous royal family. Later, Buddhism prohibited all types of consanguineous marriages when it was found that consanguinity was harmful to the offspring or the next generations due to inbreeding.

- **Consanguineous Marriage in Christianity and Judaism:** The attitude of Christianity and Judaism toward kinship is based on the book of Leviticus. The book of Leviticus states that "none of you shall approach any one of his close relatives to uncover nakedness. I am the Lord" (Leviticus 18:5). This statement is interpreted differently by different religious groups. For example, the Jews interpret it and permit first-cousin and uncle-niece marriage. In contrast, the attitude of Christians toward consanguinity is not uniform. The Orthodox Church interprets it firmly and prohibits consanguineous marriage. In contrast, the Latin church prohibits marriage with a biological relative up to and including a third cousin, and the Roman Catholic Church requires diocesan permission for marriage between cousins (Bittles et al. 2001; White 2009).

Discourse of Consanguinity on Autism

This volume addresses an anthropological study of consanguineous marriages, which is underpinned by the modern medical focus on managing the genetic risk of autism among the offspring. This study explored the effects of genetic risk on the progeny due to the consanguineous marriage of their parents. This study suggests that the risk is "high," applies to all consanguineous marriages, and equates to "cause" and "doubling" the background risk. Risk discourse is frequently also a vehicle for social and economic agendas. This volume invites readers to ask themselves to discourage consanguineous marriages to protect future generations from autism and other genetic diseases (Shaw and Raj 2011).

There is heterogeneity in formal medical provisions for managing risk and in how consanguineous couples and intermarrying communities perceive and negotiate the implications of risk information (ibid). Sometimes, people calculate risk in unexpected ways that do not correspond with the bilaterality of Mendelian genetics. However, as in South Asia, particularly in Bangladesh, it reflects a local understanding of closeness in patrilineal kinship through consanguineous marriage. These accounts contribute to the knowledge concerning how genetics and kinship ties are interlocked in consanguineous marriage and thus affect autism spectrum disorders.

Concluding Remarks

Consanguineous marriage or cousin marriage is a type of interfamilial union, defined as the marriage between two blood-related individuals who are second cousins or closer. Over a billion people live in communities where consanguineous marriage is a traditional and respected sociocultural and biological trend of marital union. The primary reasons for preference for consanguineous marriage in communities with high consanguinity rates include maintaining the lineage, solidarity of family, relative ease for the partners in finding a suitable spouse, backing the female status and improved relationships with in-laws, lowering the marital cost, reducing the custom of dowry, enhancing the likelihood of getting better care for people in old age, and above all better stability of marital relationship. These factors seem to carry more significance in the context of protective and semi-protective cultures of many Middle Eastern, South Asian, West Asian, and sub-Saharan African societies.

References

Aggarwal, P. C. (1976). "Kinship and Marriage among the Meos of Rajasthan." In Imtiaz Ahmed (ed.). *Family, Kinship, and Marriage among the Muslims in India.* New Delhi: Manohar.

Akrami, S. M., V. Montazeri, S. R. Shomali, R. Heshmat, and B. Larijani. (2009). "Is there a Significant Trend in the Prevalence of Consanguineous

Asperger, H. (1944). "Die 'Autistischen Psychopathen' Im Kindesalter." Archiv furr Psychiatrie and Nervenkrankheiten, (117): 76-136

Bennett, R., A. Motulsky, and A. Bittles. (2002). "Genetic Counseling and Screening of Consanguineous Couple and their Offspring: Recommendations of the National Society of Genetic Counselors." *Journal of Genetic Counseling,* (11): pp. 97–119.

Bhende, A., and T. Kanitkar. (1982). *Principles of Population Studies.* Bombay: Himalaya Publishing House

Bindu, P. S., S. Desai, K. E. Shehanaz, M. Nethravathy, and P. K. Pal. (2006). "Clinical Heterogeneity in Hallervorden-Spatz Syndrome: A Clinicoradiological Study in Thirteen Patients from South India." *Brain Development,* (28):343–7.

Bittles A. (2023). The global prevalence of consanguinity. http://www.consang.net accessed June 2023. 11-02-2023

———. (2009). "Commentary: The Background and Outcomes of the First-Cousin Marriage Controversy in Great Britain." *International Journal of Epidemiology,* 38 (3):1453–1458.

———. (2008). "Consanguinity and Its Relevance to Clinical Genetics." *Clinical Genetics.* 60 92): pp. 89–98.

Sandridge

Bittles, A. H., and M. L. Black. (2010). "Evolution in Health and Medicine Sackler Colloquium: Consanguinity, Human Evolution, and Complex Diseases." *Proc National Academic Science*, 107 (1):1779–1786.

Buddhism and Marriage. (2014 March 19). *The Tibetan Buddhist Encyclopedia.* Accessed 02:10, February 18, 2024, from http://www.tibetanbuddhistencyclopedia.com/en/index.php?title=Buddhism_and_Marriageandoldid=145165.

Bundey, S., H. Alam, A. Kaur, S. Mir, and R. J. Lancashire. (1990). "Race, Consanguinity and Social features in Birmingham Babies: A basis for a Prospective Study." *Journal Epidemiol Community Health*, (44): pp. 130–135.

Cambell, J. M. (2006). Autism Spectrum Disorder. In (Eds.) by R. W. Kamphaus and J.M. Campbell in *Psychodiagnostic Assessment of Children*. New Jersey: John Willey and Sons.

Dousset, Laurent. (2018). *Australian Aboriginal Kinship: An Introductory Handbook with Particular Emphasis on the Western Desert*. Manuels du Credo, Marseille: Pacific-credo Publications.

Hamamy, Hanan. (2012). "Consanguineous Marriage Perception Consultation in Primary Health Care Settings." *Journal of Community Genetics*, 3(3): 185–192

Hamamy, H, S. E. Antonarakis, L. L. Cavalli-Sforza, S. Temtamy, G. Romeo, L. P. Ten Kate, R. L. Bennett, et al. (2011). *Consanguineous Marriages, Pearls, and Perils*. Geneva International Consanguinity Workshop report. Genet Med, 13:841–847

Heidari, F., S. Dastgiri, and N. Tajaddini. (2014). "Prevalence and Risk Factors of Consanguineous Marriage." *European Journal of General Medicine* [serial online], 11(4):248–255.

Introduction

Hussain, R. (1998). "The Impact of Consanguinity and Inbreeding on Perinatal Mortality in Karachi, Pakistan." *Paediatr Perinat Epidemiol*, (12): pp. 370–382.

Jacobson, D. (1976). "The Evil of Virtue: Purdah and the Muslim Family in the Bhopal Region of Central India." In Imtiaz Ahmed (ed.) *Family, Kinship and Marriage among the Muslims in India.* Manohar, New Delhi.

Kanner, L. (1943). "Autism Disturbances of Affective Contact." *Nervous Child,* 4 (2): 217–250.

Kapacdia, K. M. (1966). Marriage and Family in India. New Delhi: Oxford University Press.

Kapur, P. (1974). *The Changing Status of the Working Women in India.* New Delhi: Vikas Publishing House Pvt. Ltd.

Levitt, G. (2003). Incest/inbreeding taboos. International Encyclopedia of Marriage and Family. Available at: http:// family.jrnk.org/pges/854/incest-inbreeding-Taboos-Sibling-Marriage-Human-Isolates.himil. Accessed March 28, 2015.

Magnus, P., K. Berg, and T. Bjerkedal. (1985). "Association of Parental Consanguinity with Decreased Birth Weight and Increased Rate of Early Death and Congenital Malformation." *Clinical Genetics,* (28):342–445.

Maheswari, K., and L. Wadhwa. (2016). "Role of Consanguinity in Pediatric Neurological Disorder." *International Journal of Pediatrics,* 3(3):939–942.

Maloney, C., K. M. Ashraful Aziz, and Profulla C. Sarker. (1981). *Beliefs and Fertility in Bangladesh.* Dhaka: ICDDRB.

"Marriage in Tehran? A Review of Three Generations". *Journal of Genetic Counseling, 18*(1):82–6.

Mirza, Abul-Fazl. (1924). Sayings of the Prophet Muhammad. Allahabad: Allahabad Reform Society

Modell, B. and A. Darr. (2002). "Science and Society: Genetic Counseling and Customary Consanguineous Marriage." *Nature Reviews Genetics*, 12 (3):225–229.

Mumtaz, G., H. Tamin, and M. Kanaan. (2007). "Effect of Consanguinity on Birth Weight for Gestational Age in a Developing Country." *American Journal of Epidemiology*, (165):742–752.

Nalini, A., N. Gayathri, T. C. Yasha, S. Ravishankar, A. Urtizberea, and K. Huehne. (2008). "Clinical, Pathological and Molecular Findings in two Siblings with Giant Axonal Neuropathy (GAN): Report from India." *Europe Journal of Medical Genetics*, (51):426–35.

Obeidat, B. G., Y. S. Khader, Z. O. Amarin, M. Kassawneh, and M. AlOmari. (2010). "Consanguinity and Adverse Pregnancy Outcomes: the North of Jordan Experience." *Maternal Child Health Journal*, 14 (2):283–9.

Ottenheimer, Martin. (1996). *Forbidden Relatives: The American Myth of Cousin Marriage*. Illinois: University of Illinois.

Prayson, A. S. (2016). "Autism, Genetics and Inbreeding: An Evolutionary View." *Journal of Public Health and Epidemiology*, 8(5):67–71.

Paul, Diane B., and Hamish G. Spencer. (2008). "'It's OK, We are Not Cousins by Blood': The Cousin Marriage Controversy in Historical Perspective." *PLOS Biology*, 6 (12):2627–30.

Sarker, Profulla C. (2017). *Social Structure and Fertility Behavior: A Cross-Cultural Study*. Dhaka: Mother's Publication.

———. (1997). *Social Structure and Fertility Behavior: A Cross-Cultural Study*. Dhaka: Center for Development Services.

———. (2015). "Consanguinity, Inbreeding, and Their Impact on Reproductive Health and Human Development in Inbred Communities." *The Indian Journal of Anthropology*, 3 (2): 69–80.

Schulpen, T. W., J. C.Wieringen, P. J. Brummen, J. M. Riel, F. A. Beemer, P. Westers, and J. Huber. (2006). "Infant Mortality, Ethnicity, and Genetically Determined Disorders in the Netherlands." *European Journal of Public Health*, 16 (1):291–294.

Shaw, Alison, and Aviad Raz. (2011). *Cousin Marriage between Tradition and Genetic Risk and Cultural Change*. Oxford: Berghahn.

Sindh, Kausal K. (1974). *Family Planning: The Religious Factors.* New Delhi: Abhinav Publishers.

Stoltenberg, C., P. Magnus, R. T. Lie, A. K. Daltveit, and L. M. Irgens. (1997). "Birth Defects and Parental Consanguinity in Norway." *American Journal of Epidemiology*, (145): 439–448.

Tadmouri, G. O., P. Nair, T. Obeid, M. T. Al Ali, N. Al Khaja, and H. A. Hamamy. (2009). "Consanguinity and Reproductive Health among Arabs." *Reproductive Health*, 8 (6):17–23.

Yunis, K., G. Mumtaz, and F. Bitar. (2006). "Consanguineous Marriage and Congenital Heart Defects: A Case-Control Study in the Neonatal Period." *American Journal of Medical Genetics Part A*, (140): 1524–1530.

White, S. W., and R. Roberson-Nay. (2009). "Anxiety, Social Deficits, and Loneliness in Youth with Autism Spectrum Disorders." *Journal of Autism and Developmental Disorders*, 39 (2): 1006–1013.

White, S. W. (2009). "Anxiety in Children and Adolescents with Autism Spectrum Disorders." *Clinical Psychology Review*, 29 (3): 216–229.

Chapter 2

METHODS AND TECHNIQUES APPLIED TO CONDUCT RESEARCH

Introduction

The research method is an umbrella concept for a research project, which covers selecting the research setting, literature review, developing the theoretical framework, and identifying the specific and general objectives of the research and the population under study. In addition, it includes the sampling procedure applied to select the study population. The research questions, along with the expected result of the research, are considered in the methods. Besides, the research design is also incorporated in the methods because research design is the blueprint of the entire research project, which focuses on personnel (e.g., workforce) that must carry out the research project within a specific schedule and estimated budget. The main thrust is to apply the methods and techniques for collecting primary and secondary data, editing, and processing data, analyzing data using the different quantitative and qualitative methods and strategies, and finally, writing procedures for the research report.

Theoretical Framework

The theoretical framework of this study is confined to four main concepts: cousin marriage, consanguinity, inbreeding, and autism. The word *consanguineous* comes from the Latin words *con*, meaning "shared," and *sanguine*, meaning "blood." Consanguinity describes a relationship between two people who share an ancestor or common blood. Different populations across the globe favor such marriages, and usually, they are bound to traditional customs, beliefs, and values to keep their property in a united form within the family.

Cousin marriage has deep historical origins, and it was permitted and practiced within ancient Israel, Greece, and Palestine. It was not prohibited in the early Hebrew or Christian religion, and it predated the rise of Islam (Tillion 1983). Anthropologist Tillion (1983) links it with the rise of settled agriculture, strengthening ties between kin who held land in standard and perpetuating gender norms that promote female seclusion and dependence on men. She argues throughout the ancient Mediterranean world that the most desirable marriage came to be defined as "marriage with a very close relative belonging to own lineage" (Tillion 1983). Rather than exchanging women, the idea became to keep all the girls in the family for the boys. This cultural ideal has emotional and psychological consequences for gender roles and female dependency on men.

On the other hand, inbreeding describes the mating between two blood relatives, i.e., consanguineous relatives; the degree of inbreeding is usually measured as the coefficient of inbreeding. The value of this coefficient is equal to the probability that an individual will have inherited alleles of a gene that are "identical by descent," the same form of an allele inherited from a single common ancestor. The coefficient is of medical significance when considering autosomal recessive conditions and genetic load (Bittles 2001). The phenomenon by which the number of individuals affected by autosomal recessive disorders increases due to inbreeding. Inbreeding is used to create inbred strains of rats and mice (typically requires twenty generations of inbreeding) that are genetically identical. Members of the inbred stain can be genetically altered commonly by knocking out or changing a single gene to observe its effect. They have provided a significant deal of information about the function of specific genes.

Autism is associated with inbreeding due to consanguinity. Autism is a complex neuro-behavioral condition that includes impairments in social interaction and developmental language and communication skills combined with rigid, repetitive behaviors. Because of the range of symptoms, this condition is now called autism spectrum disorder (ASD). Symptoms of autism typically appear during the first three years of life and may continue lifelong. Some children show signs from birth. Others seem to develop normally at first, only to slip suddenly into symptoms when they are eighteen to thirty-six months old. On the other hand, autism is a developmental disorder characterized by impaired social interactions and restricted or repetitive patterns of behavior. However, the condition is often missed and not diagnosed until later in a child's life, especially when the condition is mild or moderate or even in severity.

A large proportion of children with autism, between 50 and 70 percent, have additional learning disabilities, i.e., an IQ lower than 70. In contrast, such disabilities are absent in the remaining children, who are often described as high functioning. For some children, language is limited or lacking altogether. For others, speech can be fluent, but even so, their use of language to communicate in social contexts is odd, awkward, and often one-sided. Stereotyped and inflexible behavior ranges from hand flapping and finger-twisting to idiosyncratic special interests (e.g., the ins and outs of drainpipes).

In recognition of this heterogeneity, researchers frequently use the term autism spectrum disorder (ASD) to describe the different variants of autism, including pervasive developmental disorder-not otherwise specified (PDD-NOS) and Asperger syndrome (Wing 1996). The latter is diagnosed in children with no apparent language delay, though the distinction between Asperger syndrome and high-functioning autism is somewhat blurry. Under these circumstances, researchers have acknowledged that a complete understanding of autism is required, including multiple scientific perspectives, viz. genetics or biology, cognition, and behavior (Frith et al. 1991). In addition to interactions with the environment, there is likely to be a complex interplay between these explanatory levels. For example, abnormalities in early cognitive development could have profound secondary effects on later brain and psychological development. Likewise, the premise of early behavioral intervention is that it should capitalize on the plasticity of the developing brain to alter underlying abnormal brain processes. It has been found in family studies that autism is mainly genetic, though the identification of specific genes is proving more difficult than

Methods and Techniques Applied to Conduct Research

initially anticipated, mainly due to the disorder's heterogeneity (Bolton et al. 1994; Folstein and Rutter 1977). Research suggests that multiple interacting genes are involved in their inheritance (Pickles et al. 1995) and that the neurobiological abnormalities are pervasive and not confined to any brain region (Belmonte et al. 2004).

Psychologists have focused their efforts on the cognitive level of explanation to identify the underlying processes that might account for the various behavioral manifestations of the disorder. Historically, and in the interests of parsimony, the emphasis upon these theories has been to posit a single primary cognitive deficit that could explain the development of autism. Theories from three cognitive domains have dominated the field:

(a) Theory of Mind: The ability to reason about the mental states of others.
(b) Executive Control: A set of abilities necessary for flexible behavior in novel circumstances.
(c) Central Coherence: The natural propensity to process information in context.

More specifically, autism is a developmental retardation that is characterized by isolation, cognitive shortcomings, language difficulties, and self-tantrums, which start before thirty months of age in different stages of the life of the offspring.

Objectives of the Study

The main objective of this research is to examine to what extent cousin or consanguineous marriages may cause the offspring to become autistic through inbreeding with the gene mutation of the same genetic pole or same blood group. The specific objectives of this study are as follows:

- To know the marital background of the couple, whether they are involved in a marital tie, either cross-cousin or parallel-cousin marriage.
- To explore the socioeconomic status of the parents and their offspring, including the parents' age structure, level of education

and occupation, family types and authority structure, and the gender-specific age of the autistic children.
- To find out the reasons given for the preference of consanguineous marriages.
- To examine what extent cousin or consanguineous marriages may affect the offspring to be autistic in inbred communities.
- To explore the treatment procedures applied by parents for the treatment of their autistic children.

Research Questions

All the research questions are based on the study's objectives. The following research questions will clearly explain the study's focus.

- What are the leading causes behind the interest in consanguineous marriages?
- How does it affect autism for the offspring through gene mutation as well as inbreeding?
- How do parents apply the treatment procedures for their offspring?

Expected Results

- The expected results of the research project are the quasi-economic and quasi-sociocultural interests involved in either cross or parallel-cousin marriages.
- A significant percentage of autism is higher among the children whose parents are involved in marital ties, either cross-cousin marriage or parallel cousin marriage, compared to the parents who were not engaged in marital ties in cousin marriage.
- Inborn diseases like autism may occur due to various degrees of consanguinity and inbreeding. In the system of consanguineous marriage, gene circulation is confined within the kin group or the genetic pool itself. Consequently, the same genetic trade is compelled to distribute and redistribute genes among several generations, ultimately destroying the original gene structure and leading to autism among the offspring.
- Autism may be demonstrated in speaking style or by a failure to understand social rules or consequences of behavior, lack of

curiosity and difficulty solving problems, decreased learning ability and ability to think logically trouble remembering things, and an inability to meet educational demands required by the school.

Sampling Procedure

A stratified purposive sampling procedure was used here to select the study population, aiming to focus in-depth research findings on relatively small and representative sizes of autistic children and their parents. About one hundred autistic children were selected from the different stratified groups of parents. This stratification is identified based on socioeconomic conditions in terms of sources of income, occupation, education, social status, and so on.

Samples were chosen because of the size of the population of this research. The controls in such samples are usually identified as representative areas and representative characteristics of an individual's age, sex, marital status, and socioeconomic status in terms of the level of education, occupation, family types, and authority structure to explore the process of making decisions about autistic children. Purposive stratified sampling differs from stratified random sampling in that the actual selection of the units to be included in the sample in each group was done purposively rather than by random method (Dawodu et al. 2005).

Research Design

The research design includes six special education schools for autistic children in Dhaka, which were identified to select the study population. About one hundred autistic children were selected based on a stratified purposive sampling procedure, and two parents were chosen accordingly. The estimated schedule of the research project was about twelve months. About nine persons in different positions were involved in 60.5-man months to conduct the research.

- **Setting of Research**: Dhaka City was selected as the research area for this research project because most special education schools are concentrated in Dhaka City to provide special education for autistic children. The six special education schools for autistic children were selected using purposive sampling. Moreover, it was chosen to get easy access to the special education institutes for the collection of primary data about autistic children and the consanguineous marital background of their parents, which includes sociocultural and quasi-economic interests behind the cross-cousin and parallel cousin marriage. Most mothers of autistic children were found to be well-educated and very conscious and enthusiastic in providing information about their children. Under these circumstances, the setting of this research project was appropriate for getting accurate and reliable information about personal and sensitive subjects.

- **Population of the Study**: The study population was 100 (one hundred) autistic children aged 5–12 years and their 200 (two hundred) parents. A stratified purposive sampling method was applied to select one hundred autistic children irrespective of ethnicity, religious affiliation, and gender identity and their two hundred parents as the population of this research. The autistic children were selected considering their level of education, age, gender, and nature of autism. It also includes the parents' marital status about consanguinity and the quasi-economic, sociocultural, and political reasons. Complete enumeration was conducted to collect in-depth qualitative data.

- **Field Investigators and Supervisor**: Four field investigators and one supervisor were selected through intensive interviews to collect data for five months; all have graduate-level education in the social science field. Two days of intensive training were given along with the one-day field demonstration before going for data collection. They were responsible for data collection through face-to-face interviewing and administering a questionnaire. In addition, they were also responsible for collecting qualitative data using case studies, focus group discussion (FGD), key informants (KI) interviews, observation methods, and maintaining dairy for field notes.

Methods and Techniques Applied to Conduct Research

Methods of Data Collection

Several methods and techniques have been applied to collect primary data from this research project's quantitative and qualitative perspectives. These are (1) a survey using a questionnaire, (2) observation of both participants and non-participants, (3) a focus group discussion (FGD), (4) a case study, and (5) a critical informant interview.

- **Survey Method:** The survey was conducted using a questionnaire administered either to the mothers or fathers of the selected autistic children. A cross-sectional survey was conducted of all members using a questionnaire.

- **Observation Method:** The observation method was applied during data collection, either by interviewing using a questionnaire or during an FGD or KI interview, by watching the gestures and posture of the informant's recollection of accurate information. In addition, active participant and passive participant observation methods were also applied during data collection.

- **Focus Group Discussion Method:** The focus group discussion (FGD) method was also used to collect data from a holistic perspective from a group of people. Usually, each FGD consisted of eight to ten parents of autistic children. The researchers acted as facilitators and rapporteurs. The FGD method was applied to keep the study's objectives in view.

- **Case Study Method:** The case study method was used to collect in-depth information on the rephrase of the study. The case was selected considering the socioeconomic background of the parents of the autistic children. The field investigators spent hours together collecting data from the selected cases.

- **Use of Key Informants:** The key informants were used to supplement the survey data. They were selected from a cross-section of people (viz., schoolteachers, maidservants, peer groups, professionals, marriage registrars, and so on) who were directly or indirectly associated with the problems.

Data Editing: The research associate carefully edited the data before processing it. Sometimes, he visited the research area for reinvestigation when he found areas for improvement in the previous information.

Data Processing: In data processing, emphasis is usually given to cross-data processing between two variables. The collected data was processed using both quantitative and qualitative techniques.

Data Analysis: Data was analyzed using quantitative and qualitative methods and techniques. Although emphasis has been placed on qualitative techniques based on fact, quantitative methods still need to be used in data analysis. Quantitative methods were used to analyze data based on figures to supplement the qualitative analysis in graphs and pie to strengthen the qualitative study.

Research Report

In many ways, a research report can be considered a summary of the research process that highlights the background of the research, methods, and techniques applied for data collection, research findings, recommendations, and other vital issues in detail. It is a well-written research report that provides all the information the readers need about the core areas of the research project. This research report is reliable because the researchers have taken the utmost care in conducting the research project and is a true testimony of all the work done to garner the specificities of the research (Sarker 2020). The researchers have already applied some of the basic features for writing this research report, which are given below:

- It is a detailed presentation of research processes and findings, including tables and graphs.
- It is written in standard and lucid language so the readers can easily understand.
- This research report has been written focusing on the third person.
- It is informative and based on first-hand verifiable information.
- It is formally structured with headings, sections, and, to some extent, bullet points.
- It always includes policy implications for the future of action.

Outlines of Research Report

Most scientific research reports, regardless of discipline and type of research, require a framework. A report is a structured piece of writing designed to present findings or recommendations to a specific audience. A good report has a clear structure and is written in sections with subheadings. There are many ways that an academic report might be structured, depending on the task the researchers have set (Yong 1996).

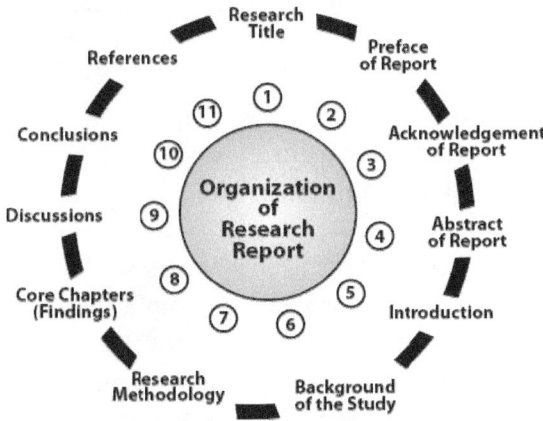

Fig. 2: Outlines of a Report

Concluding Remarks

In concluding remarks, the concept of research methods is the strategies, processes, and techniques that have already been utilized in the collection of both qualitative and quantitative data and analysis to uncover new information on consanguinity, inbreeding, and their effects on autism spectrum disorders (ASD) in the inbred community of Dhaka metropolitan city. Although it is a small-scale study, and as a result, it is difficult to generalize the findings at the societal level, the depth of the study is significant for plans of action to prevent and reduce ASD in avoiding consanguineous marriages through genetic counseling.

References

Anderson, C., K. Day, and P. McLaughlin. (2006). "Mastering the Dissertation: Lecturers' Representations of the Purposes and Processes of Master's Level Dissertation Supervision." *Studies in Higher Education,* 31(2): 149–168.

Camp, W. G. (2001). "Formulating and Evaluating Theoretical Frameworks for Career and Technical Education Research." *Journal of Vocational Educational Research,* 26(1): 27–39.

Dawodu, A., L. Al-Gazali, E. Varady, M. Varghese, K. Nath, and V. Rajan. (2005). "Genetic Contribution to High Neonatal Lethal Malformation Rate in the United Arab Emirates." *Community Genetic,* (8): 31–34.

Eisenhart, M. (1991). "Conceptual Frameworks for Research Circa 1991: Ideas from a Cultural Anthropologist; Implications for Mathematics Education Researchers." Proceedings of the Thirteenth Annual Meeting North American Paper of the International Group for the Psychology of Mathematics Education. Virginia: Blacksburg.

Iqbal, J. (2007). "Learning from a Doctoral Research Project: Structure and Content of a Research Proposal." *The Electronic Journal of Business Research Methods,* 5(1):11–20.

Lester, F. (2005). "On the Theoretical, Conceptual and Philosophical Foundations for Research in Mathematics Education". *ZDM,* 37(6): 457–467.

Lovitts, B. (2005). "How to Grade the Dissertation." *Academe,* 91(6): 18–23.

Luse, A., B. Mennecke, and A. Townsend. (2012). "Selecting a Research Topic: A Framework for Doctoral Students." *International Journal of Doctoral Studies,* 7 (2):143–152.

Lysaght, Z. (2011). Epistemological and Paradigmatic Ecumenism in "Pasteur's Quadrant:" Tales from Doctoral Research. Official

Conference Proceedings of the Third Asian Conference on Education in Osaka, Japan.

Melendez, J. (2002). "Doctoral Scholarship Examined: Dissertation Research in the Field of Higher Education Studies." Unpublished Dissertation.

Merriam, S. (1997). "Qualitative Research and Case Study Applications in Education." San Francisco: Jossey-Bass.

Miles, M. B., and A. M. Huberman. (1994). *Qualitative Data Analysis: An Expanded Source Book*. Newbury Park: Sage Publications.

Munhall, P., and R. Chenail. (2008). *Qualitative Research Proposals and Reports: A Guide*. Sudbury, MA: Jones and Bartlett.

Sarker, Profulla C. (2022). *Paradigms of Qualitative Research in Multidisciplinary Perspective*. Bhairab: Sheik Hasina University of Science and Technology.

———. (2020). *Research Project Proposal across the Disciples: Guide to Writing Research Project Proposal*. Dhaka: Royal University of Dhaka.

———. (2021). *Paradigms of Case Study: An In-depth Quest*. Dhaka: Royal University of Dhaka.

Torraco, R. J. (1997). *Theory-Building Research Methods*. In Swanson R. and E. Holton III (Eds.), Human Resource Development Handbook: Linking Research and Practice. San Francisco: Berrett-Koehler.

Trifiletti, L., A. Gielen, D. A. Sleet, and K. Hopkins. (2005). "Behavioral and Social Sciences Theories and Models: Are They Used in Unintentional Injury Prevention Research?" *Health Education Research*, 20(3): 298–307.

Yong, P. V. (1996). *Scientific Social Survey and Research*. New Delhi: Prentice-Hall.

Chapter 3

CONSANGUINEOUS MARRIAGES IN CROSS-CULTURAL PERSPECTIVE

Introduction

Conventionally, marriage is matrimony or wedlock in the sociocultural union as well as a legal contract between two or more opposite sex of people, which is recognized as husband and wife that establishes rights and obligations between spouses and their children (Haviland et al. 2011; Grant and Bittles 1997). Many cultures have already practiced and continue to practice marriage between relatives to strengthen family ties and retain property within the family or among the relatives involved in kinship ties (Hussain and Bittles, 2000). Different studies have revealed that consanguineous marriages are usually socioculturally motivated and can be genetically harmful. Studies also revealed that the consequences of consanguineous marriages and inbreeding are considerable social science, genetics, and health science concerns. Mating of relatives leads to increased genetic homogeneity of inbred individuals due to similarities between contributing paternal and maternal genetic characteristics. The detrimental effects of inbreeding are the consequence of homozygosis of harmful genes and thus may affect the offspring with autism and other health problems.

It has been found in different studies that the offspring of consanguineous parents have higher rates of congenital malformation along with other health hazards. Inbreeding and consanguinity are used interchangeably to describe unions between couples. Inbreeding in population genetics refers to a departure from nonrandom "mating" in that individual's "mate" with those more genetically similar. Inbreeding is a pejorative term when applied to human beings because of its negative impact on society and the health system, and the coefficient of inbreeding (F) is used in population genetics to describe this phenomenon (Bennett et al. 2002).

Studies revealed that at least one of every five marriages is consanguineous between couples who are second cousins or closer in the Middle East and North Africa, and the rate is higher than 50 percent in some parts of the world. Consanguineous marriage generates serious health problems like autism for the offspring and constitutes an economic problem with medical costs and thus affects human capital. The prevalence of consanguineous marriages and the resultant kinship networks can shape various dimensions of society, ranging from institutional structure to attitudes such as trust, individualism, and nepotism (Hermelin and O'Connor, 1970).

Consanguineous Marriage in Regionality

The variations in legislative and religious rules are also reflected in the prevalence of consanguineous marriage across regions from a cross-cultural perspective. In the Western world, consanguineous marriages constitute less than 1 percent of marriages, but this practice remains widely prevalent in many other places. The estimates range from 30–50 percent in Middle Eastern countries, 20–40 percent in North Africa, and 10–20 percent in South Asia (Maian and Mushtaq 1994; Bittles 1998; Bittles 2001). There is also significant variation within countries. In India, for example, the National Family Health Survey 1992–93 (IIPS and ORC Macro International 1995) reveals that 16 percent of marriages are consanguineous; this varies from 6 percent in northern India and 36 percent in the southern parts of India (Banerjee and Roy 2002: 22). Some research reports also suggests that the practice of consanguineous marriage is growing in popularity in Western countries, particularly in migrant communities mainly who migrated from Middle East, North Africa, and South Asia where the Muslim population is numerically dominated (Bittles 2001; Hoskin and Powel 1985).

Consanguinity in Cross-Cultural Perspective

Consanguinity is rooted in blood relation, derived from the Latin word *consanguinity*, which is the property of being from the same kinship as another person. In that aspect, consanguinity is the quality of being descended from the same ancestor as another person. Consanguineous marriage is frequent in many populations. It has been recently estimated that consanguineous couples make up about 6.7 billion people globally (Jain 2011).

There is wide diversity in the attitudes of the different major world religions and philosophies toward consanguinity. In general terms, consanguineous marriage is permitted within Judaism, in some branches of Christianity, Islam, Dravidian Hinduism, and Buddhism. However, the prevalence of a specific type of marriage is allowed and may vary according to the precepts and traditions of each religion and denomination; in some cases, these characteristics appear to have altered significantly through time. In all major religions, there are also communities whose marriage practices are at variance within the majority's customs, beliefs, and values, in some cases suggesting a carry-over from earlier times and systems of worship, which are cited here. The practice of consanguineous marriage of the major religions is cited here.

- **Consanguinity in Islam:** Consanguineous marriage is widely favored by most Muslims worldwide. According to recent estimates, the resident Muslim population of India is over one hundred million. However, apart from a few numerically small or geographically defined surveys, little is known about their patterns of marriage preferences since the partition of the Indian Subcontinent in 1947. This study seeks to determine the prevalence and patterns of consanguineous marriages contracted among Indian Muslims at regional and state levels during the last two generations (Hussain 1998). Data from the 1992 and 1993 Indian National Family Health Survey (NFHS) were used in the analysis. The NFHS was a nationally representative survey of ever-married women aged 13–49 years conducted across twenty-five states of India. Overall, 22 percent of marriages were found to be contracted between spouses related as second cousins or closer, ranging from

15.9 percent in the eastern states to 32.9 percent in the western states of India. In all parts of the country, first-cousin marriages were the preferred form of consanguineous union, and in four of the five regions, paternal first-cousin marriages predominated. Despite predictions to the contrary, there was no evidence of a significant change in the prevalence of consanguineous unions throughout the study period, which extended from the late 1950s to the early 1990s.

Consanguineous marriage has had considerable attention as a causative factor in the prevalence of genetic disorders. Iran, with its majority Muslim population, has a high rate of consanguineous marriage. In Iranian tradition, first-cousin marriage is an acceptable and appreciated custom. However, there seems to be no encouragement of consanguineous marriage in the Islamic context; it is merely mentioned as a traditional and common custom (Dawodu et al. 2005).

Cousin marriages, including those between first cousins, are permitted by Islamic law and scriptures and were practiced by Prophet Hazrat Muhammad and his companions. His practice of cousin marriage, in addition to cementing the practice's legality, renders the practice a *sunnah*, or a good deed worthy of commendation, given his status as *al-insan al-kamal* (the perfect man). Cousin marriages have been common throughout Islamic history and remain so in Muslim-majority nations today, comprising a significant percentage of the total population of these nations.

Prophet Hazrat Muhammad married his cousin Zaynab binte Jahsh who, in addition to being the daughter of Umaimah binte Abd al-Muttalib (a sister of Muhammad's father), was also the former wife of his adopted son, Zayd ibn Harith. The marriage proved immensely controversial, not because Zaynab and Muhammad were cousins—cousin marriages were fairly common throughout much of the ancient world—but because Zaynab had previously been married to Muhammad's adopted son. The controversy was of such scale that Muhammad ultimately produced a revelation in the Quran addressing the matter, absolving him of any proposed guilt.

- **Consanguinity in Hinduism:** It is already noted in the introduction of this book that proscriptions on consanguinity within Hinduism vary between the North and the South of India. In the Aryan Hindu tradition of North India, marriage between relatives is usually prohibited (Kapadia 1958). For example, early Indian economic historiography describes marriage within the Hindu caste system in North India as one in which a man is obliged to marry outside his family but within the caste and usually within the sub-caste to which his family belongs. A family consists of persons reputed to be descended from a common ancestor and between whom marriage is prohibited (Anstey 1952: 48). This tradition prohibits marriage to relatives for seven generations on the male side and for five generations on the female side (Balasubramaniam 2002). On the other hand, the South Indian, or Dravidian Hindu tradition, permits consanguineous marriages (Balasubramaniam 2002; Epstein 1973; Reddy 1993; Vatuk 1982). For example, one form of marriage common among Tamils in South India is the gift of marriage of a girl to a suitable person from her maternal uncle or paternal aunt's family. The preponderance of consanguineous marriage in South India is also reflected in popular parlance in the Tamil language; a wife is expected to address her husband traditionally, not by using his first name, but by calling him *athan*, which is the Tamil word for "father's sister's son." Similarly, the Tamil word for mother-in-law is *Mamiya*, which translates to "brother's sister's wife." This illustrates that consanguineous marriage has been common in South India (Balasubramaniam 2002). This is also reflected in the average distance migrated by a woman at the time of marriage. This distance exceeds twelve miles in rural North India but less than eight miles in rural South India (Reddy 1993). Overall, it is believed that religion may contribute to the prevalence of consanguinity in some parts of the world, yet it is not the primary driving force of this practice. The religious sanctions and prohibitions around this practice are also quite diverse and have changed over time.

- **Consanguinity in Christianity:** Under Roman civil law, the early canon law of the Catholic church, couples were forbidden to marry if they were within four degrees of consanguinity. In the ninth century, the church raised the number of prohibited degrees to seven and changed how they were calculated. This meant that the nobility struggled to find marriage partners as the pool of non-related prospective spouses became smaller. They had to defy the church's position or look elsewhere for eligible marriage candidates. In 1215, the Fourth Lateran Council made what they believed was a necessary change to canon law, reducing the number of prohibited degrees of consanguinity from seven back to four. The method of calculating prohibited degrees was also changed: Instead of the former practice of counting to the common ancestor and then down to the proposed spouse, the new law computed consanguinity by counting back to the common ancestor. In the Roman Catholic Church, unknowingly marrying a closely consanguineous blood relative was grounds for a declaration of nullity. However, during the eleventh and twelfth centuries, dispensations were granted with increasing frequency due to the thousands of persons encompassed in the prohibition at seven degrees and the hardships this posed for finding potential spouses (Brundage 2009). After 1215, the general rule was that while fourth cousins could marry without dispensation, the need for dispensations was generally significantly reduced (Brundage 2009). In fourteenth-century England, for example, papal dispensations for annulments due to consanguinity were relatively few (Helmholtz 2007).

The connotation of the degree of consanguinity varies by context. However, most cultures define a degree of consanguinity within which sexual interrelationships are regarded as incestuous or the "prohibited degree of kinship."

- **Consanguinity in Buddhism:** Buddhism originated in North India in the third century BC, and the prince Buddha is reputed to have married his first cousin. Perhaps for this reason, there is no overall proscription of consanguineous marriage within the Buddhist tradition. In Buddhism, marriage is not a religious obligation, a means for procreation, or a romantic notion of love.

It is simply an option for everyone to make. If individuals believe marriage will bring them happiness and keep them enlightened, they are free to choose. Buddhism allows each person to decide whether they want to be married, how many children they want to have, and to whom they want to marry. Buddhism does not provide rules about marriage. The philosophy of Buddha offers advice to help a person live happily within a marriage. This advice is thought to help people to get a chance at a happy romantic relationship. In Buddhist text, the Buddha believed that the biggest hurdle in marriage is spousal weakness for other partners. He saw the weakness and trouble that other romantic interests can contribute to making a happy family.

Consanguineous Marriages in Bangladesh

Bangladesh is the eighth most populous country in the world and one of the most densely populated nations. The total population of Bangladesh is about 165 million; among them, about 90.4 percent are Muslim. Of the rest, 8.5 percent are Hindu, 0.6 percent are Buddhist, 0.4 percent are Christian, and the rest of 0.1 percent are others, respectively. The different religious groups have different attitudes toward consanguineous marriages in Bangladesh. In Islam, consanguineous marriages are allowed, and it is practiced among Muslims in Bangladesh. On the other hand, consanguineous marriage is strictly prohibited among the Hindus. This prohibition has continued for approximately seven generations from the male side and five generations from the female side (Kapadia 1958). After the specific generation is over, they are allowed to get married within the distant or kin group, which may be called endogamous marriage or the marriage of the same caste or clan in the extended lineage of the distant kinship relations.

The practice of consanguineous marriages is expected in the Muslim community worldwide (Tayebi et al. 2010). Islam allows consanguineous marriages but always discourages first-cousin marriages (Bittles 2008). In Bangladesh, very few studies have attempted to determine the current prevalence of consanguinity and its effects on genetic disorders like autism among the offspring. It has been reported that the prevalence of consanguineous marriage in Bangladesh is 6.6 percent (Oniya et al. 2019).

In Buddhism, all types of consanguineous marriages are strictly prohibited. No one is allowed to be involved in consanguineous marriage. The attitude of Christianity toward consanguinity is not uniform. Consanguineous marriages are flexible in Christianity from the perspective of different churches. The Orthodox Church prohibits consanguineous marriage, while the Latin Church prohibits marriage with a biological relative up to and including a third cousin. On the other hand, the Roman Catholic Church requires permission from the priest for marriage between cross and parallel cousins (Bittles et al. 2001).

Consanguineous marriage is considered one of the predisposing factors for genetic diseases in Bangladesh. Consanguinity increases the prevalence of genetic and congenital anomalies among offspring (Anwar et al., 2020). Different studies reveal a higher risk of recessive genetic disorders among children of consanguineous parents.

Bangladesh is one of the Muslim-dominant countries in South Asia, and consanguineous marriages are practiced among Muslims. However, the prevalence, causal factors, and genetic and reproductive consequences were not studied thoroughly. The necessity of population-based surveys to compare the frequency of disorders in children of consanguineous couples with non-consanguineous parents was not studied intensively in Bangladesh. Several studies have suggested that first-cousin marriage is the most favored type among Muslims because of the quasi-economic interests of both parties. However, the prevalence of consanguineous marriages may differ among geographic origins where the economy is land-based and agricultural, and the tendency is increasing toward agro-based industry. It is revealed in many small-scale studies that patrilineal consanguineous marriages are preferred in peasant society compared to matrilineal in Bangladesh.

In the past few decades, Bangladesh has experienced a noticeable increase in education among girls. On the other hand, the expansion of urbanization and rural-urban migration is also increasing. As a result, the tendency among the younger generation to form a nuclear family also grows immediately after the wedding ceremony. Consequently, partner selection is shifting from the parents' choice to the choice of the bride and the groom. Under these circumstances, the probability of consanguineous marriages declines. It should be noted that the agrarian economy and customary practice of consanguineous marriages are associated with the deep-rooted culture in terms of customs, beliefs, and values among the Muslims in Bangladesh.

Types of Consanguineous Marriage

Consanguinity is defined as the marriage between individuals with a common ancestor, which is also mentioned in the previous chapters of this volume. This section deals with the types of consanguineous marriages among the parents of autistic children under the research population of the project. About one hundred spouses were selected whose children were found autistic, and they were involved in either parallel cousin or cross-cousin marriages or non-cousin marriages.

Parallel cousin marriage is divided into two categories: paternal parallel-cousin marriage and maternal parallel-cousin marriage. In paternal cross-cousin, marriage is solemnized between the father's brother's son and the father's brother's daughter (Fa et al. Da). On the other hand, the maternal parallel cross-cousin marriage happens between the father's sister's daughter (Fa Si Da) and the mother's sister's son (Mo et al.). In addition, cross-cousin marriage is divided into two categories: patrilateral cross-cousin and matrilateral cross-cousin (Sarker 2017). Patrilateral cross-cousin marriage occurs between the father's sister's daughter (Fa Si Da) and the mother's brother's son (Mo et al.). Similarly, matrilateral cross-cousin marriage is solemnized between the mother's brother's son (Mo et al.) and the mother's sister's daughter (Mo Si Da). A model of different types of consanguineous marriages, along with the symbols of kinship ties, is enclosed here to get a clear idea of how consanguineous marriages occur among the parents and thus affect the autism of their offspring (Sarker 2017).

Symbols of Kinship Relations

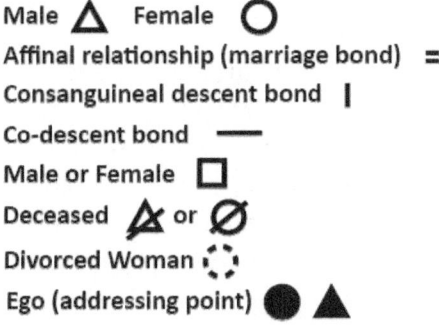

The above symbols identify the network kinship relationship among the people of a family, whether they are related to consanguineal or affinal relationships. This kinship tie contributes to studying the family structure from a cross-cultural perspective (Sarker 1917). It also contributes to the readers' knowledge of how the human relationship is formed and identifies using the kinship terminology based on the respective language. A model is given below to understand the different types of consanguineous marriage among spouses whose children are found autistic.

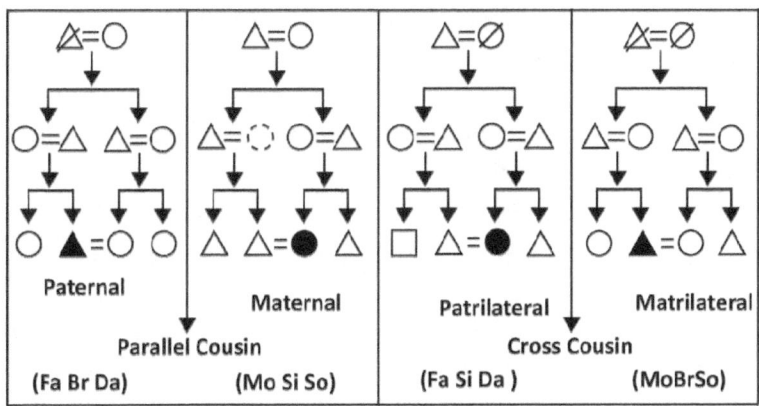

Fig. 3: Model of Different Types of Consanguineous Marriage among the Spouses of 114 Autistic Children

It is found in this study that about 60 percent of parallel cousin marriages, either paternal or maternal cross-cousin, were solemnized among the parents of the autistic children, and 40 percent were involved in cross-cousin marriage, either patrilateral or matrilateral cross-cousin marriages.

Among parents involved in parallel-cousin marriages, about 78 percent were in paternal parallel-cousin marriages, and 22 percent were in maternal parallel-cousin marriages. It should be noted that spouses preferred paternal parallel-cousin marriage to maternal parallel-cousin marriage to keep their property within their own families, which is associated with the quasi-economic interest of the bride and groom and their parents. It is revealed that less preference was given to maternal parallel cousin marriage because the property may transfer to other families, but their social ties may remain intimate. On the other hand, about 65 percent of patrilateral cross-cousin was found among the parents compared to 35 percent in matrilateral cross-cousin marriages. It indicates that most of them belong to a patriarchal social structure where male domination is still predominating as a deep-rooted culture.

According to the principles of Mendelian theory of genetics, consanguineous marriages confer an elevated risk that a child will have autism as a recessively inherited genetic disease (Modell and Darr 2002). A recessive condition is caused by inheriting two copies: one from each parent of a gene mutation that in a single copy carries no significant health risk. If two people carry the same recessive mutation, their risk of having an affected child is 25 percent. Two biologically unrelated people have a chance of about 2–3 percent of both being carriers of the same gene mutation, but for first cousins, this risk increases to approximately 4–6 percent because they have a grandparent in common from whom they might inherit the same gene (Grant and Bittles 1997).

Reasons for Consanguineous Marriage

The reasons for preference for consanguineous marriages are primarily both parties' quasi-social and quasi-economic interests (Sarker 2017). This research project has already identified the following specific reasons for consanguineous marriages.

- Enforces couple stability and compatibility.
- Better relationship with in-laws.
- Renew and strengthen family ties.
- Enforces family solidarity.
- Transmission and continuity of cultural values.

- Keep property within the family.
- Understanding of hidden health problems.
- Possibility of fewer dowries for weddings.
- Less possibility of marital dissolution in terms of desertion, separation, and divorce.
- Opportunity to get a daughter living nearby to get support in a crisis.

In communities with high consanguinity rates, sociological studies indicate that consanguineous marriages will enforce the couples' stability due to higher compatibility between husband and wife who share the same social relationships after marriage as before marriage, as well as compatibility between the couple and other family members, especially those involved in kinship ties.

It has been observed that consanguineous marriages are more favorable for women's status, including the wife's better relationship with her in-laws, who can support her in times of need. Usually, it is believed that marrying within the family reduces the possibilities of hidden uncertainties in health and financial issues. It is also thought that consanguinity strengthens family ties and enforces family solidarity. In addition, cousin marriages provide excellent opportunities for transmitting cultural values among newly wedded couples and their continuity (Sandridge et al. 2010). Premarital negotiations regarding marriage financial matters are more easily conducted and sometimes less costly. It is revealed that the wife's parents prefer to have their daughter living near them and enjoy their grandchildren's presence. Moreover, wealthy landowners prefer to keep their property within the family through marriages within the kin structure (Bittles 2008).

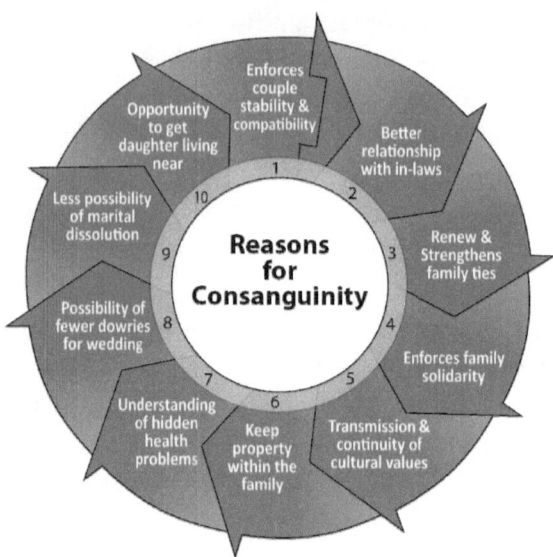

Fig. 4: Model on Reasons of Consanguinity

Concluding Remarks

The third chapter of this book discusses the prevalence of consanguineous marriage, which is practiced from a cross-cultural perspective in this study. The parents involved in parallel cousin marriage found that about 78 percent were paternal parallel cousin marriages, and 22 percent were maternal parallel cousin marriages. It should be noted that spouses prefer paternal parallel cousin marriage to maternal parallel cousin marriage because they want to keep their property within their own families, which is associated with the quasi-economic and quasi-social interest of the bride and the groom as well as their parents. It is revealed in this study that most of the couples were unaware of the genetic risk of consanguineous marriage for their future generation; instead, they thought about the immediate socioeconomic benefit of both parties.

References

Baldwin, J. W. (1994). *The Language of Sex: Five Voices from Northern France Around 1200*. Chicago: University of Chicago Press.

Banerjee, S. K. and T. K. Roy. (2002). "Parental Consanguinity and Offspring Mortality: The Search for Possible Linkage in the Indian Context." *Asia-Pacific Population Journal*, 17(1): 17–38.

Bittles, A. H. (2001). "Consanguinity and Its Relevance to Clinical Genetics." *Clinical Genetics*, 2 (60): 89- 98.

———. (1994). "The Role and Significance of Consanguinity as a Demographic Variable." *Population and Development Review*, 4 (5): 561–584.

Brundage, James A. (2009). *Law, Sex, and Christian Society in Medieval Europe*. Chicago: University of Chicago Press.

Dawodu, A., L. Al-Gazali, E. Varady, M. Varghese, K. Nath, and V. Rajan. (2005). "Genetic Contribution to High Neonatal Lethal Malformation Rate in the United Arab Emirates." *Community Genetic*, (8): 31–34.

Fatema, K., T. Das, A. Mannan, and S. M. Zaman. (2017). "Frequency Distribution of Congenital Anomaly and Associated Maternal Risk Factors." *Mymensingh Medical College Journal*, 26 920:658–66.

Grant, J. C., and Bittles, A. H. (1997). "The Comparative Role of Consanguinity in Infant and Childhood Mortality in Pakistan." *Annals of Human Genetics*, 61(1):143–9.

Helmholz, R. H. (2007). *Marriage Litigation in Medieval England*. Cambridge: Cambridge University Press.

Hermelin, B., and N. O'Connor. (1970). *Psychological Experiments with Autistic Children*. Oxford: Pergamon Press.

Hoskin, G., and R. Powel. (1985). *Chronic Childhood Disorder*. Bristol: John Wright and Sons Ltd.

Hussain, R. (1998). "The Impact of Consanguinity and Inbreeding on Perinatal Mortality in Karachi, Pakistan." *Paediatric Perinatal Epidemiology*, (12): pp. 370–382.

International Institute of Population Sciences, Mumbai, and ORC Macro International (1995). National Family Health Survey 1992–93. Mumbai: IIPS

Jain, S. (2011). "Consanguinity and Inherited Epilepsies." *Neurology Asia*, (16): pp. 11–12.

Kapadia, K. M. (1958). *Marriage and Family in India*. Calcutta: Oxford University Press.

Maian, A., and R. Mushtaq. (1994). "Consanguinity in Population of Quetta (Pakistan): A Preliminary Study," *Journal of Human Ecology* 5 (3): 49–53.

Sarker, Profulla C. (1917). *Marriage, Kinship, and Family: Biosocial Network System*. Dhaka: Mother's Publications.

Shieh, J. T. C., A. H. Bittles, and L. Hudgins. (2012). "Consanguinity and the Risk of Congenital Heart Disease." *American Journal of Medical Genetics*, 158A (3): pp. 36–41.

Teeuw, M. E., L. Henneman, Z. Bochdanovits, P. Heutink, D. J. Kuik, and M. C. Cornel. (2010). "Do Consanguineous Parents of a Child Affected by an Autosomal Recessive Disease Have More DNA Identical-by-Descent Than Similarly Related Parents with Healthy Offspring? Design of a Case-Control Study." *BMC Medical Genetics*, 11 (3):1–5.

Verma, I. C., and S. Bijarnia. (2002). "The Burden of Genetic Disorders in India and a Framework for Community Control." *Community Genet*, 5 (1):192–6.

World Health Organization. (2013). "Birth Defects in Southeast Asia: A Public Health Challenge: Situation Analysis." WHO: *Southeast Asia Journal of Public Health*, 34 (2): 68–75.

Chapter 4

SOCIODEMOGRAPHIC PROFILE OF THE PARENTS AND THE AUTISTIC CHILDREN

Introduction

Social demography deals with questions of population composition and change and how they interact with sociological variables at the individual and contextual levels. Social demography also uses demographic approaches and methods to make sense of social, economic, and political phenomena. A demographic profile combines social and demographic factors defining people in a specific group or population. In other words, when we talk about sociodemography, we mean different social and demographic features that help to understand what group members have in standard features. The socio-demographic profile includes the age structure of the spouses involved in consanguineous or non-consanguineous marriages, their level of education, family types, authority structure of the family, and occupation structure of the parents. This chapter also discusses the gender-specific age of autistic children and their categories of autism. The socio-demographic profile is a valuable tool for social scientists, public health and health care experts, policy analysts, and policymakers, as well as planners because it illustrates the problem of age and gender-specific autism trends, especially those whose parents were in consanguineous marriages. The gender-specific age structure depicts the distribution of autistic children in various age groups of each gender.

Demographers, sociologists, social psychologists, and evolutionary biologists are highly interested in the mechanism responsible for these sociodemographic changes in a population of individuals. In research, sociodemographic characteristics of a population or individual have been essentially investigated to provide a correlated understanding of a particular phenomenon. For instance, lifestyle diseases, disease occurrences, disease severity, and susceptibility are correlated in medical research (Trent and South 1992; Ramirez et al. 1993; Kravdal 2002; Skrzypczak 2009). However, it is a philosophical tradition that sociodemographic features accompany population research (Thomas et al. 2006). Despite this philosophy, description, and judgment of the population or individual's socio-demographic characteristics are primarily based on frequencies and percentages, odds ratio, and cluster statistics.

Age Structure of Parents

Age is one of the most critical sociodemographic factors influencing people's decisions. Typically, people within the same age group or category have shared experiences, affecting their preferences. A graph is given here to get a clear idea about the ages of the parents of the autistic children (Sarker 2020). It is revealed in Graph 1 that the age of the wife is lower compared to the husband among the selected couples whose children were autistic. It is also found that about 40 percent of husbands and 30 percent of wives are aged 35–39. On the other hand, 13 percent of husbands and 14 percent of wives belong to the age group of 25–29, and 4 percent of husbands and 9 percent of wives belong to the age group of 20–24, respectively. Similarly, 15 percent of husbands and 10 percent of wives belong to the age group of 40–44, and only 5 percent of husbands and 3 percent of wives belong to the age group of 45 years and above. Interestingly, the husbands preferred younger wives in their conjugal life to get maximum service.

Sociodemographic Profile of the Parents and the Autistic Children

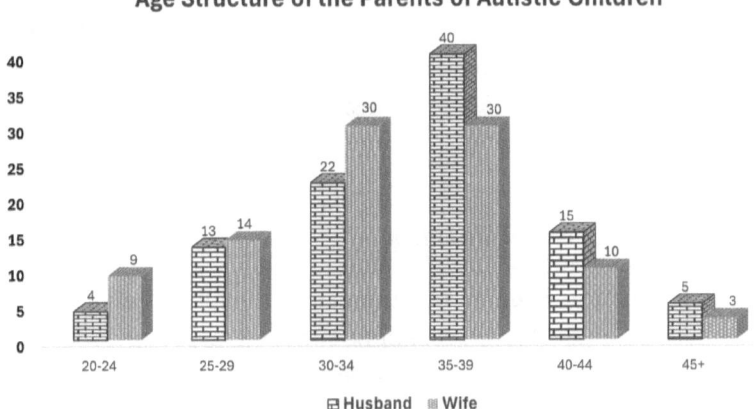

Graph 1: Age Structure of the Parents of Autistic Children

Level of Education of Parents

The spouse's level of education is sometimes an indicator of the kinds of jobs they do and how much they earn. In many communities, higher levels of education mean better employment opportunities and more income. Having this at the back of anyone's mind can align their core messaging with the different realities resulting from parents' educational backgrounds. More specifically, the education level means the number of years of schooling—for example, high school graduates, college graduates, university graduates, or any other advanced education. A graph is enclosed here to show the level of education of the parents of autistic children.

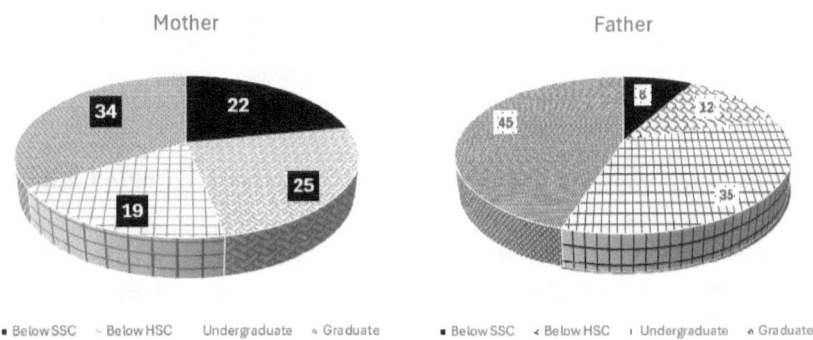

Graph 2: Level of Education of the Spouses of Autistic Children

Graph 2 shows that 45 percent of the fathers had graduated compared to 34 percent of the mothers of autistic children. About 8 percent of fathers and 22 percent of mothers had school-level education, i.e., below the Secondary School Certificate (SSC). It is interesting to note that all the parents were found to be educated.

Occupation Structure of Parents

Occupational structure refers to the aggregate distribution of occupations in society, defined by skill level, economic function, or social rank. Various factors influence the occupational structure, including the economy's structure, technology and bureaucracy, the labor market, business and status, and prestige. More specifically, the occupational structure of the parents of autistic children refers to the percentage of their workforce involved and employed in various economic ventures. In other words, the number of working parents employed in different sectors, including household activities, can be identified from the occupational structure. A graph of occupation structure for parents of autistic children is given here.

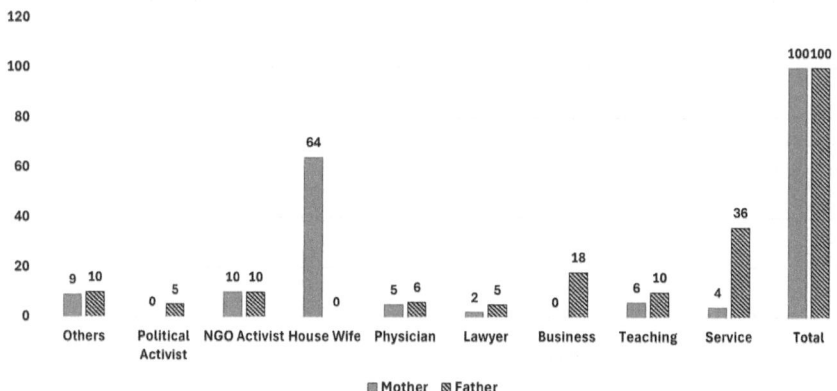

Graph 3: Occupation Structure of the Parents of Autistic Children

The above graph reveals that about 36 percent of the autistic children's fathers were service holders compared to 4 percent of their mothers. In addition, the second-largest number of fathers were involved in business. On the other hand, 64 percent of mothers were engaged in household activities. This indicates that a significant percentage of mothers were involved in taking care of their autistic children and their household activities.

Family Types of Autistic Children

The family, on account of its smallness and intimacy and the constant demands its members make on each other as a whole person, is a small community within itself, within which relationships are bound to be both intense and ambivalent: involving love but also hate; fulfillment of demand but also restriction; relaxation and confidence. A family is responsible for caring for its aged members and any of its members suffering from illness, accident, or misfortune. It consists of allocating a pattern of rights and duties defining the area of life concerned with marital, parental, and domestic relationships (Sarker 2017). The concept of family is rooted in developing many kinds of network relationships, such as conjugal, parental, and filial relationships. All relationships are based on kinship ties. A graph is stated here to provide a clear idea about the distribution of autistic children's family types and the authority structure of those families.

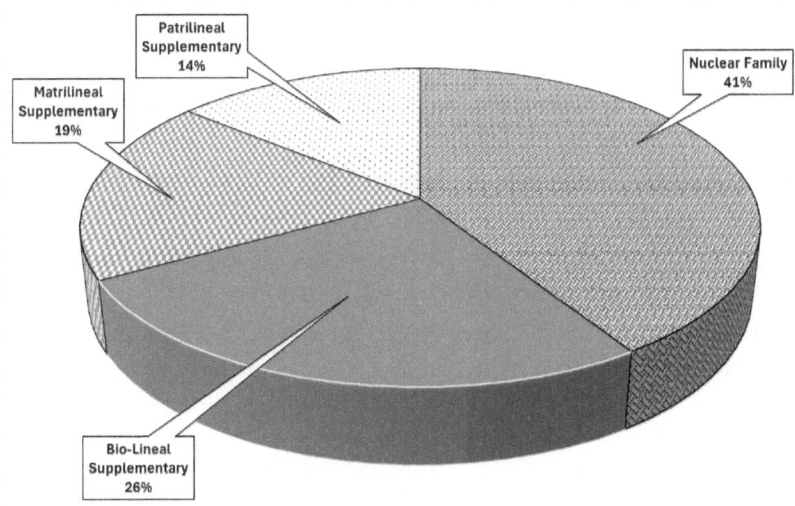

Pie 01: Family Types of Autistic Children

The type of family depends upon the composition of its membership pattern in kinship ties, which also varies from one society to another or even in the different segments of the same society. Moreover, the type of family is not a static phenomenon. Instead, it is dynamic due to factors like birth, death, marriage, desertion, separation, divorce, and migration of its members. For example, the death of a husband or wife in a nuclear family changes its original type from nuclear to a subnuclear family, or the marriage of a son in an atomic family transforms it into a joint family. The family is divided into joint or extended family and nuclear family (Aziz 1979).

Authority Structure of Family

Family authority depends on the family's structure, composition, and function. It is vested in the person who takes responsibility for the maintenance of the family and plays a dominant role in decision-making in any affair of the family irrespective of sex, either individually (husband or wife) or jointly (both husband and wife). Thus, the concept of authority undertakes to assign *power* to the family. The authority structure of the family is divided into three categories: (a) patriarchal, (b) matriarchal, and (c) egalitarian (Sarker 2017).

- **Patriarchal Authority Structure:** In the patriarchal authority structure, the family's authority is vested in the father or any responsible elder male member. He is the sole authority to make decisions on any matter related to the family. No one is allowed to share or interfere in making the decision. Under these circumstances, the decision of any family affair is in the hands of the father or, in the absence of the father, any responsible elder male member, and the decision is always unilineal.

Sociodemographic Profile of the Parents and the Autistic Children

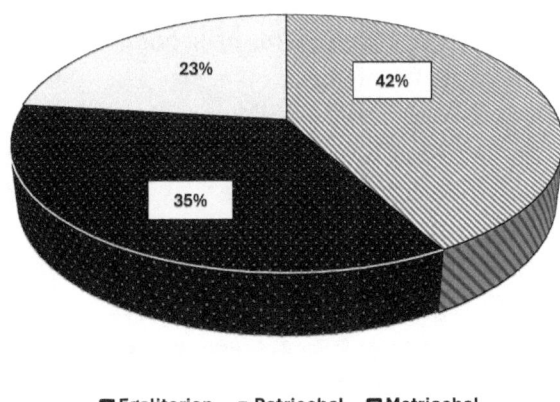

◨ Egalitarian ▪ Patriachal ◻ Matriachal

Pie 02: Autistic Children in Authority Structure of Families

- **Matriarchal Authority Structure:** In matriarchal authority, the mother or any responsible older female member of the family decides any matter of the family in the absence of a male member or if the male member is inactive. This usually happens when the wife owns the parent's property or the property of her previous husband or is the earning member of the family. Here, the power or authority of the family is associated with the economy.
- **Egalitarian Authority Structure:** In the egalitarian authority structure, the husband and wife share equal or roughly equal responsibility in decision-making about any family affair. This usually happens when both the husband and wife are educated and earning members of the family (Sarker 2017).

A graph is given here to get a clear idea about the distribution of autistic children in the authority structure of families where autistic children live. It is revealed in Pie 2, named autistic children in authority structure of families, that about 35 percent of autistic children live in the patriarchal authority structure of families. On the other hand, 23 percent of families were found to have a matriarchal authority structure. It was found that 42 percent of families were egalitarian authority structures. The tendency of egalitarian authority structure family is increasing in urban settings compared to rural ones.

Gender-Specific Age of Autistic Children

Age structure means the composition of a population in terms of the proportions of individuals of different ages. The gender-specific age structure of autistic children is the distribution of autistic children in gender perspectives of various ages. It is a valuable tool for social scientists, public health and healthcare experts, policy analysts, and policymakers because it illustrates the problem of age and gender-specific autism trends, especially those whose parents were in consanguineous marriages (Imaizumi 1986). The gender-specific age structure depicts the distribution of autistic children in various age groups for each gender. A graph is enclosed here to give a clear idea of this context.

Gender-specific age structure reflects the proportions of autistic children at different stages of age about their gender identity. These variables are important indicators of children's status, and they can be used to explore how many of them are the offspring of consanguineous or non-consanguineous couples. A graph is given here to get a clear idea about the age and gender of autistic children and the marital status of their parents, either consanguineous or non-consanguineous marriage.

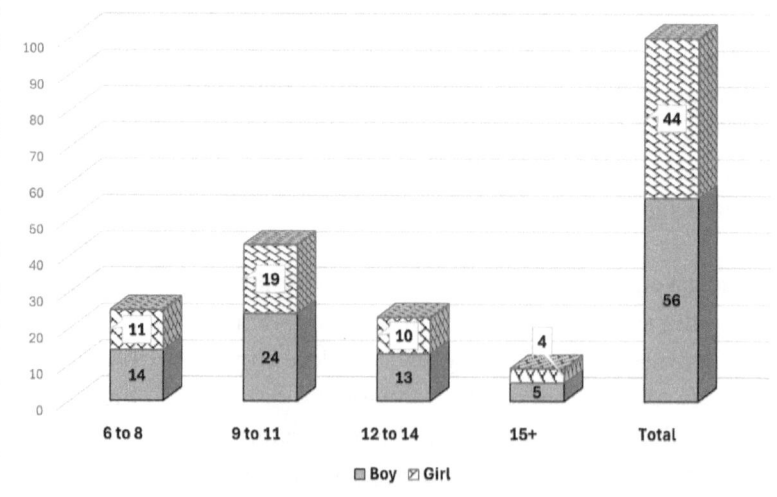

Graph 4: Gender-Specific Age Structure of the Autistic Children.

It is revealed in graph no. 4 that 25 percent of autistic children belonged to the age group of 6–8 years, and among the 14 percent were boys, and the remaining 11 percent were girls. On the other hand, 43 percent of autistic children belonged to the age group of 9–11 years; 24 percent were boys, and the rest of the 19 percent were girls. About 23 percent of autistic children belonged to the age group of 12–14 years, and among them, 13 percent were boys and 10 percent were girls. Only nine percent of children were older than 14 years. It is interesting to note that the number of boys is higher compared to girls who are victims of autism.

Categories of Autism Spectrum Disorders

There are three categories of autism spectrum disorders, namely a) mild autism b) disorder, c) moderate autism disorder, and c) acute autism disorder, which are given in the following graph 5. All these disorders have been explained here to provide explicit knowledge.

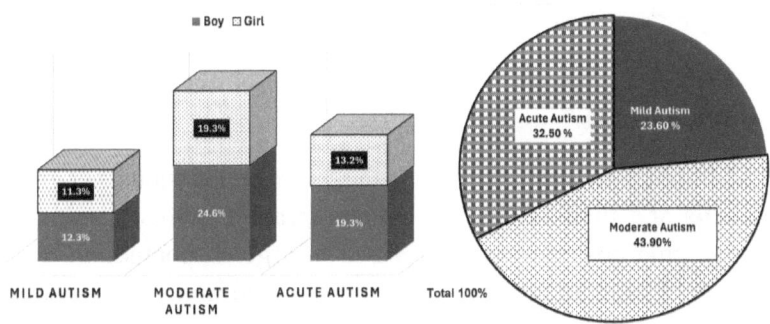

Graph 5: Categories of Autistic Children

a) **Mild Autism Disorder:** This is sometimes called atypical autism. In mild autism, the children usually have fewer and milder symptoms than those with autistic disorder. The symptoms might cause only social and communication challenges. It is revealed in graph number 5 that about 23.7 percent of children were autistic. Among them, 12.3 percent were male, and 11.3 percent were female. This category of autistic children requires minor support to lead an everyday life.

b) **Moderate Autism Disorder:** In moderate autism disorder, people with Asperger syndrome usually have milder symptoms of autistic disorder. They might have social challenges and unusual behaviors and interests. However, typically, they do not have problems with language or intellectual disability. About 43.9 percent of autistic children were found with moderate autism disorder. Among them, 24.6 percent were boys, and the rest of 19.3 percent were girls. This category of autistic children requires substantial support to lead a productive life.

c) **Acute (severe) Autism Disorder**: In severe autism, the disorder is what most people think of when hearing the word "autism." Children with this autistic disorder usually have significant language delays, social and communication challenges, and unusual behaviors and interests. Many children with this autistic disorder also have intellectual disability. About 32.5 percent of autistic children were found to have severe autistic disorder. About 19.3 percent were boys, and the rest of 13.2 percent were girls. They do require exhaustive support to survive.

Concluding Remarks

Sociodemographics describe the relationship between individuals or groups of individuals and their attained sociodemographic statuses, including sociodemographic positions and successes in a given population over a given period. Sociodemographic statuses are common, universal, and desirable positions, achievements, and advantages every individual strives and competes to attain, achieve, maintain, and upgrade, which is influenced by the biological and social environments, driven and regulated by a continuum of competitions through genetic, physiological, demographic, and psychosocial competition, and selectively evolved through the mechanism of genetic, physiological, demographics, psychosocial selection, and resultant psychosocial fitness and sociodemographic evolution.

References

Aziz, K. A. M. Ashraful. (1979). *Kinship in Bangladesh*. Dhaka: ICDDR, Bangladesh.

Kravdal, Ř. A. (2002). "Cancer Survival Model That Takes Sociodemographic Variations in Normal Mortality into Account: Comparison with Other Models." *Journal of Epidemiol Commun Health*, 56 (2): 309–18.

Ramirez, A. J., K. L. Pinder, M. E. Black, M. A. Richards, W. M. Gregory, & R. D. Rubens. (1993). "Psychiatric Disorders in Patients with Advanced Breast Cancer: Prevalence and Associated Factors." *European Journal of Cancer*, 29(4): 524–7.

Sarker, Profulla C. (2020). *Paradigms of Case Study in Multidisciplinary Perspective: An In-Depth Quest*. Dhaka: Center for Research, Knowledge Management, and Human Resource Development, Royal University of Dhaka.

———. (2022). *Paradigms of Qualitative Research in Multidisciplinary Perspective*. Bhairab: Sheikh Hasina University of Science and Technology.

———. (1917). *Marriage, Kinship, and Family: Biosocial Network System*. Dhaka: Mother's Publications.

———. (2017). *Social Structure and Fertility Behavior in Bangladesh: A Cross-Cultural Study*. Dhaka: Mother's Publications.

Skrzypczak, M., P. Łaski, U. Czerniak, and W. Kycler. (2009). "Do Chronological Age and Selected Sociodemographic Factors Affect the Quality of Life in Females with Breast Cancer?" *Anthropological Review*, 72 (2): 31–44.

Trent, K., & S. J. South. (1992). "Sociodemographic Status, Parental Background, Childhood Family Structure, and Attitudes toward Family Formation." *Journal of Marriage and the Family 1992*, 54(2): 427–439.

Chapter 5

SIGNS AND SYMPTOMS OF AUTISM SPECTRUM DISORDERS (ASD)

Introduction

Autism spectrum disorder (ASD) is a neurological and developmental disorder that affects how people interact, communicate, learn, and behave with each other. Although autism can be diagnosed at any age, it is described as a "developmental disorder" because symptoms generally appear in the first two years of life (Baranek 1999; Bassili et al. 2000). However, the condition is often missed and not diagnosed until later in a child's life, especially when the condition is mild or even severe. Many factors might contribute to the incidence of autism. For example, it is often difficult for a child with autism to be appropriately diagnosed, as pediatricians are relatively inexperienced in the diagnosis and management of psychiatric disorders compared to their Western counterparts. In general, fewer psychiatrists specialize in childhood development problems in Bangladesh. The lack of awareness among parents regarding ASD, including a failure to recognize symptoms and seek diagnosis and treatment, is also likely to be a factor, especially in cases of children suffering from mild forms of autism. So, both under-diagnosis and under-reporting may play a vital role in the disparity in the prevalence of autism between the East and the West (Dover and Le 2007).

Evidence of Autism Spectrum Disorders

Autism spectrum disorder (ASD) is a pervasive developmental disorder characterized by impairments in social interaction, communication, and restricted, repetitive, and stereotyped behaviors. Symptoms of individuals with ASD can range over a wide variety of combinations of these three core behavioral deficits, with severities ranging from mild to severe. In addition, individuals with ASD are likely to exhibit a variety of comorbid disorders, including mental retardation, phobias, and depression (Matson and Nebel-Schwalm, 2007). Therefore, each person with ASD has a unique combination of symptoms, symptom severities, and comorbid disorders—furthermore, these symptoms and characteristics of children with ASD change with age and development.

It is estimated that worldwide, about 1 in 100 children have autism (Lewis 2009; Tadmouri et al. 2009). This estimate represents an average figure and reports evidence that varies substantially across studies. A recent estimate by Bangabandhu Sheikh Mujib Medical University (BSMMU) confirmed that almost 2 in 1000 children have autism in Bangladesh, where the evidence is much higher in urban areas compared to rural settings. There is a greater consensus among learned communities that the more an individual knows about autism, the better inclusive environment they can create for autistic children. Therefore, autism is a challenging task for human resource development. Under the circumstances, a nationwide awareness program needs to be initiated to discourage people from getting into consanguineous marriages, which is one of the genetic causes of autism in the offspring.

Sing and Symtoms of ASD

Autism spectrum disorder (ASD) is a neurodevelopment disorder characterized by social communication deficits, restricted or repetitive behaviors, and stereotyped interests. The onset of ASD symptoms or behaviors can occur in one of two ways: Early or regressive (Goin-Kochel et al. 2015; Boterberg et al. 2019). In early onset, ASD symptoms (e.g., deficits or delay in social and speech development) occur in the first year of life. Children with regressive onset initially exhibit typical development. However, in the second or third year of life, they begin to exhibit ASD symptoms or behaviors accompanied by the loss of previously established social, communicative, and motor skills (Goin-Kochel et al., 2015). Researchers have proposed a third onset pattern, plateau, in which children display typical development patterns in the first year, followed by a slowdown or lack of further development. Although children retain previously acquired skills in plateau onset, their development plateaus with no progress to advanced skills such as language or joint attention (Bauman 2010; Lintas and Persico 2009).

Individuals with ASD may be at risk for deficient cognitive abilities, sensory processing anomalies, impaired language development, and other medical conditions (e.g., seizures, sleep disorders, and psychological disorders) (Schaefer 2016). Researchers have continued to study the cause of ASD, as findings have the potential to inform ASD diagnosis, treatment, management, and prognosis, help predict or anticipate possible comorbid medical conditions, and increase adherence to intervention and rehabilitation regimens. Furthermore, parents of children with ASD often support ASD etiological research as it helps with family planning and reduces the guilt and anxiety parents feel that is associated with their speculations as to the cause of their child's ASD (Bölte et al. 2019).

Autism spectrum disorder (ASD) is a developmental disability caused by differences in the brain. People with ASD often have problems with social communication and interaction and restricted or repetitive behaviors or interests. People with ASD may also have different ways of learning, moving, or paying attention. It is important to note that some people without ASD might also have some of these symptoms. However, for people with ASD, these characteristics can make life very challenging. Autism spectrum disorder (ASD) can manifest as different symptoms in different children. The average age of diagnosis is two years, though some children may be detected at around the age of five years. The symptoms to look out for in children with autism disorder are as follows:

- Delayed milestones.
- A socially awkward child.
- The child who has struggled to interpret.
- The child who has trouble with verbal and nonverbal communication.

Signs and Symptoms of Autism Spectrum Disorders (ASD)

Delayed Milestones: A delay in reaching language, thinking, and social or motor skills altogether is called developmental delay. Things like heredity, pregnancy complications, or premature birth can cause it. The cause is only sometimes known. Children reach developmental milestones at their own pace, and some move faster than others. Every child starts cooing, rolling over, babbling, smiling, pointing, and sitting up at an expected age. These are called milestones. Though every child grows at their own pace, the parents must visit the pediatrician if their child does not grow at their own pace. The signs and symptoms are delayed at the pace of milestones are as follows:

- The child does not smile by the age of six months.
- The child has no facial expressions by the age of nine months.
- The child has not made cooing noises or babbled by twelve months.
- No pointing or waving by the age of twelve months.
- The child does not speak by the age of sixteen months.

Signs of Social Awkwardness: Social awkwardness in children typically refers to a range of behaviors and challenges in social situations that may make it hard for them to connect with others. This could include having trouble initiating conversations, not picking up on social cues, or feeling anxious in group settings. Let us look at the signs of a socially awkward child. The parents must be concerned if their child shows signs of social awkwardness, which include the following:

- Avoids eye contact while feeding them.
- Prefers to play alone, e.i. Individualistic in nature.
- Does not respond to their name.
- Does not like being touched.
- Prefers fixed routines; even a minor change may upset them greatly.
- Has trouble understanding feelings or talking about them.

A Child Who Has Struggled to Interpret: The autistic child struggles to express their views like happiness, sadness, or anger toward others. It can be observed and understood through the following symbolic expression:

- Needs to understand how the child's facial expressions express happiness, sadness, or anger.

- The tone of voice, the way someone speaks, whether loud, soft, excited, or irritated, can convey a lot about their emotions. Children who struggle to understand these nuances might not respond appropriately to what is said.

- Body language, from crossed arms to a relaxed posture, can reveal much about someone's feelings. Children who struggle to interpret body language might miss important information about responding to or engaging with others.

Verbal and Nonverbal Communication: Verbal communication uses language, words, sentences, and voice as the medium. It involves getting a message across using sounds, words, and languages.

Nonverbal communication uses body language, facial expressions, tone, and pauses in speech as the medium. Think about it: a lie is visible in the eye, nervousness can be gauged from shaking hands or legs, and happiness is easily understood from the tone someone uses when speaking.

When people are talking to someone face-to-face, they tend to use both verbal and nonverbal communication at the same time. Most people use both verbal and nonverbal communication every day of their lives. Please think of the last conversation they had with someone. What was spoken aloud, and what was conveyed using nonverbal cues? They can develop at least one prominent verbal and nonverbal communication example. Problems of verbal and nonverbal communication of the child on the following issues:

- The autistic children keep repeating words over and over (echolalia).
- They talk in a flat tone, devoid of expressions.
- They do not understand emotions (anguish or sarcasm) in a conversation.
- They have difficulty communicating what they want.

Importance of Red Flags: In clinical terms, there are a few absolute indicators, often referred to as red flags, that identify the behavioral or developmental markers suggesting the need for further evaluation. For a parent, these red flags should be a catalyst prompting developmental

Signs and Symptoms of Autism Spectrum Disorders (ASD)

screening to ensure the child is on the right path. If the child shows two or more of these signs, he needs to ask a pediatric healthcare provider for an immediate evaluation. It is also highly recommended that whenever a parent suspects such concerns, they should go through a referral process to ensure that the child gets help.

- **Regression of Milestones:** If a child develops the milestones as expected age but loses them by 12–18 months and stops smiling, cooing, pointing, etc., it is a definite reason for concern.

- **Stimming:** If a child shows certain repetitive behaviors, such as head flapping, twitching of the eyelid, twirling, flapping their hands, or spinning in circles, they must consult the pediatrician immediately.

- **Abnormal Eating Behavior:** An abnormal desire to eat something not regarded as food, such as dirt, clay, ice, or hair. In addition, eating only certain food types, such as sweet or salty food or only yellow or a particular-colored food, is also included in abnormal eating behavior.

- **Temper Tantrums:** These are seen in kids between two and five. The child may be overly agitated, banging their head against the floor. Under the circumstances, they may have unusual reactions to harmless smells and voices.

Causes of Autism Spectrum Disorders

Autism spectrum disorder ASD) has no single known cause; instead, multiple causes are responsible. Given the complexity of the disorder and the fact that symptoms and severity may vary from individual to individual, there are probably multiple causes. There are two leading causes identified for autism spectrum disorder, viz. genetics and environment (Lewis 2009).

Genetics: Several different genes appear to be involved in autism spectrum disorder (ASD). For some children, Autism Spectrum Disorder can be associated with a genetic disorder, such as Rett syndrome or fragile X syndrome. For other children, genetic changes, i.e., mutations, may increase the risk of autism spectrum disorder. Still, different genes may affect brain development or how brain cells communicate, or they may determine the severity of symptoms. Some genetic mutations seem to be inherited, while others occur spontaneously (Becker 1999).

- **Environmental factors.** Researchers are currently exploring whether factors such as viral infections, medications or complications during pregnancy, or air pollutants play a role in triggering autism spectrum disorder ASD). These factors may be the cause or causes of autism, individually or collectively.

Characteristics of Autism Spectrum Disorders

Autism differs from person to person in severity and combinations of symptoms. There is an excellent range of abilities and characteristics of children with autism spectrum disorder. It should be noted that no two children appear or behave the same way. Symptoms can range from mild to severe and often change over time. Characteristics of autism spectrum disorder fall into two categories, viz., social interaction and Communication. Social interaction and communication problems include difficulties in normal back-and-forth conversation, reduced sharing of interests or emotions, challenges in understanding or responding to social cues such as eye contact and facial expressions, and deficits in developing or maintaining or understanding relationships (Al-Gazali and Hamamy, 2014). A child or adult with autism spectrum disorder may have problems with social interaction and communication skills, including any of the following signs:

- Fails to respond to their name or appears not to hear at times.
- Resists cuddling and holding and prefers playing alone, retreating into their world.
- Has poor eye contact and lacks facial expression.
- Does not speak, has delayed speech, or loses previous ability to say words or sentences.
- Cannot start a conversation, keep one going, or only start one to make requests or label items.
- Speaks with an abnormal tone or rhythm and may use a singsong voice or robot-like speech.

Signs and Symptoms of Autism Spectrum Disorders (ASD)

- Repeats words or phrases verbatim but does not understand how to use them.
- Does not appear to understand simple questions or directions.
- Does not express emotions or feelings and appears unaware of others' feelings.
- Does not point at or bring objects to share interest.
- Inappropriately approaches a social interaction by being passive, aggressive, or disruptive.
- Has difficulty recognizing nonverbal cues, such as interpreting other people's facial expressions, body postures, or tone of voice.

Restricted Interests and Repetitive Behavior

- Inflexibility of behavior, extreme difficulty coping with change.
- Being overly focused on niche subjects to the exclusion of others.
- Expecting others to be equally interested in those subjects.
- Difficulty tolerating changes in routine and new experiences.
- Sensory hypersensitivity (e.g., aversion to loud noises).
- Stereotypical movements such as hand flapping, rocking, and spinning.
- Arranging things, often toys, in a very particular manner.

Concluding Remarks

This chapter explores what is happening in the practice of cousin marriages in the light of genetic risk. Cousin marriages can be understood as marriages between closely related people, usually as biological kin and often as first cousins. However, "cousin" can also denote genealogically more distant kin or even a social category rather than a genealogical position. Cousin marriage is widely described in anthropological literature as the "preferred" type of marriage in many populations, mainly by Islam. It can be found in other people of different religious identities, but their number is meager. It has now also come to be widely regarded by the media and in public health discourse as genetically risky because cousin marriages are usually consanguineous to some degree. Under the circumstances, this chapter discusses the impact of consanguineous marriages on the signs and symptoms of autism spectrum disorder (ASD) of the offspring.

References

Al-Gazali, L., and H. Hamamy. (2014). "Consanguinity Dysmorphology in Arabs." *Human Heredity* (77): 93–107.

Al-Salehi, S. M. (2009). "Consanguineous Marriage in Saudi Arabia: Presentation, Clinical Correlates, and Comorbidity." *Transcult Psychiatry*, 46(2):340–347.

Baranek, G. T. (1999). "Autism during Infancy: A Retrospective Video Analysis of Sensory-Motor and Social Behaviors at 9–12 Months of Age." *Journal of Autism Development Disorder*, 29(3):213–24.

Bassili, A., S. A. Mokhtar, N .I. Dabous, S. R. Zaher, M. M. Mokhtar, and A. Zaki. (2000). "Congenital Heart Disease among Schoolchildren in Alexandria, Egypt: An Overview on Prevalence and Relative Frequencies." *Journal of Trop Pediatr.* (46):357–362.

Bauman, M.L. (2010). "Medical Comorbidities in Autism: Challenges to Diagnosis and Treatment." *Neurotherapeutics*, 7(4): 320–327.

Becker, S. (1999). "First Cousin Mating and Congenital Heart Disease in Saudi Arabia." Community *Genetics,* (10): pp. 27–121.

Bölte, S., S. Girdler, and P. B. Marschik. (2019). "The Contribution of Environmental Exposure to the Etiology of Autism Spectrum Disorder." *Cellular and Molecular Life Sciences*, 76 (4): 1275–1297.

Boterberg, S., T. Charman, P. B. Marschik, S. Bolte, and H. Roeyers. (2019). "Regression in Autism Spectrum Disorder: A Critical Overview of Retrospective Findings and Recommendations for Future Research." *Neuroscience Biobehavioral Review*, 102 (1): 24–55.

Dover, C. J., and Couteur A. Le. (2007). "How to Diagnose Autism." *Archives of Disease in Childhood*, 92 (6):540–45.

Goin-Kochel, R. P., S. S. Mire, and A. G. Dempsey. (2015). "Emergence of Autism Spectrum Disorder in Children from Simplex Families:

Relations to Parental Perceptions of Etiology." *Journal of Autism Development Disorder*, 45(3): 1451–1463.

Grant, J. C., and A. H. Bittles. (1997). *The Comparative Role of Consanguinity in Infant and Childhood Mortality in Pakistan. Annals of Human Genetics*, 61(1):143–9.

Imaizumi, Y. (1986). A Recent Survey of Consanguineous Marriages in Japan. *Clinical Genetics*, 30 (3): 230–233.

Lewis, R. (2009). *Human Genetics: Concepts and Applications*. New York: McGraw-Hill.

Lintas, C. and A. M. Persico. (2009). "Autistic Phenotypes and Genetic Testing: State-of-the-Art for the Clinical Geneticist". Journal Medical. Genetic, 9(1): 1–8.

Matson, J., and M. Nebel-Schwalm. (2007). "Comorbid Psychopathology with Autism Spectrum Disorder in Children: An Overview." *Research in Developmental Disabilities,* 28, (3): 341–352.

Schaefer, G. B. (2016). "Clinical Genetic Aspects of ASD Spectrum Disorders." *International Journal of Molecular Science*, 17(2): 180–190.

Tadmouri, G. O., P. Nair, T. Obeid, M.T. Al Ali, N. Al Khaja, and H. A. Hamamy. (2009). "Consanguinity and Reproductive Health among Arabs." *Reproductive Health*, 8 (6):17-23

Zwaigenbaum, L., M. and Penner. (2018). "Autism Spectrum Disorder: Advances in Diagnosis and Evaluation." *BMJ*, 6 (2): 361–379.

Chapter 6

CONSANGUINITY, GENE MUTATION, AND INBREEDING THEIR IMPACT ON ASD

Introduction

Cousin marriages can be understood as marriages between closely related people, usually as biological kin and often as first cousins. Still, cousin can also denote genealogically more distant kin or even a social category rather than a genealogical position. Consanguineous marriages account for 20–55 percent of marriages in the Middle East, North Africa, and Central Asia (Bittles 2012). Consanguineous marriages are also practiced by migrants from these parts of the world living in Europe, North America, and Australia. In Europe in recent years, public health debates have centered on the genetic risks and the forced nature of cousin marriages among Muslim migrants, raising concerns about the potential stigmatization of consanguineous couples and migrant communities based on their marriage patterns. Studies revealed that consanguineous marriage is related to gene mutation within the same genetic pole and thus may affect autism among the offspring of consanguineous parents. Autism is a lifelong developmental disability that affects one in social, occupational, educational, interactive, and behavioral areas (Begum and Mamin 2019). Autistic people have poor capability in determining which behaviors are considered appropriate. They carry out disruptive behaviors and experience a lack of interest in interacting with others. They have poor imagination and adaptive skills. Only a minority of adults with autism can hold a job and live independently.

Despite that, those adults are still socially vulnerable and struggle to meet the requirements of their daily lives. They are prone to experiencing anxiety and depression (The American Psychiatric Association 2013), and as a result, they are alienated from the mainstream of the population.

Consanguinity and Genetic Risk

The process of spouse selection is the medical genetic evidence that parental consanguinity increases the risk of recessive genetic problems in children. A great many medical genetic and epidemiological studies have demonstrated an association between parental consanguinity and adverse birth outcomes, mainly as pregnancy loss, which includes miscarriage and stillbirth, infant mortality, and childhood morbidity along with autism spectrum disorder (ASD) of the offspring (Bittles 2012).

There are hundreds of recessive conditions, many of which are severe or fatal and some of which are so rare that only a handful of cases have ever been reported globally. Recessive conditions can and do occur in the general population without a family history of the condition and in the absence of parental consanguinity. However, these factors make their occurrence more likely. Examining this evidence's actual and potential social impacts on the traditional process of cousin marriage is complex because it requires an engagement with diverse arenas of representation. First, understanding the basic science of genetic risk in consanguinity and the kinds of risk calculation that geneticists can make for individual couples is necessary. American Psychiatric Association (2013) described how these risks are calculated, both at the population level and in the genetic counseling of patients. Risk estimates are usually given as 4–6 percent for couples who are cousins or approximately "double" the baseline risk of 2–3 percent for an unrelated couple. However, actual risks can vary considerably, depending on the prevalence of carriers for recessive conditions in given populations, whether a couple has a family history of consanguineous marriage over generations and genetic condition. In the case of a consanguineous couple with an affected child, one should not conclude that the condition results from the parent consanguineous couple with an affected child. However, one must consider the family history of the parents.

Consanguinity

Consanguinity is the marriage between individuals with a common ancestor, as mentioned in the previous chapters. This section deals with the consanguineous marriages among the parents of autistic children under the research population of the project. About two hundred parents were selected whose children were autistic and were involved in either parallel cousin or cross-cousin marriages or non-cousin marriages. Again, parallel-cousin marriage is divided into two categories, viz. paternal parallel-cousin marriage and maternal parallel-cousin marriage. In paternal cross-cousin marriage, marriage is solemnized between the father's brother's son and the father's brother's daughter (Fa et al. Da). Similarly, maternal parallel cross-cousin marriage happens between the father's sister's daughter (Fa Si Da) and the mother's sister's son (Mo et al.).

On the other hand, cross-cousin marriage is divided into two categories: patrilateral cross-cousin marriage and matrilateral cross-cousin marriage (Sarker 2017). A patrilateral cross-cousin marriage occurs between the father's sister's daughter (Fa Si Da) and the mother's brother's son (Mo et al.). Similarly, matrilateral cross-cousin marriage is solemnized between the mother's brother's son (Mo et al.) and the mother's sister's daughter (Mo Si Da). A model of different types of consanguineous marriages, along with the symbols of kinship ties, are enclosed in chapter 3 of this volume to get a clear idea of how consanguineous marriages take place among the parents of autistic children and thus affect the autism of their offspring (Sarker 2015).

It is found in this study that about 60 percent of parallel cousin marriages, either paternal or maternal cross-cousin solemnized among the parents of the autistic children, and 40 percent were involved in cross-cousin marriage, either patrilateral or matrilateral cross-cousin marriages. Among parents engaged in parallel cousin marriages, about 78 percent were paternal parallel-cousin marriages, and 22 percent were maternal parallel-cousin marriages. It should be noted that spouses prefer paternal parallel-cousin marriage to maternal parallel-cousin marriage to keep their property within their own families, which is associated with the quasi-economic interest of the bride and groom and their parents. It has been reported that most of their spouses' parents are referred to paternal parallel cousin marriage to get socioeconomic security in their old age. It is revealed that less preference was given to maternal parallel cousin marriage because the property may transfer to other families, but their social ties may remain close and intimate. On the other hand, about 65 percent of patrilateral cross-cousin was found among the parents compared to 35 percent in matrilateral cross-cousin marriages. It seems to the author that most of them belong to a patriarchal social structure where male domination is still predominant.

According to the principles of Mendelian theory of genetics, consanguineous marriages confer an elevated risk that a child will have autism, a recessively inherited genetic disease (Modell and Darr 2002). A recessive condition is caused by inheriting two copies, one from each parent of a gene mutation that in a single copy carries no significant health risk. If two people carry the same recessive mutation, their risk of having an affected child is 25 percent (Fareed and Afzal 2014). Two biologically unrelated people have a chance of about 2–3 percent of both being carriers of the same gene mutation, but for first cousins, this risk increases to approximately 4–6 percent because they have a grandparent in common from whom they might inherit the same gene (Fareed et al. 2017)

Inbreeding

Inbreeding is a problem in humans because it heightens the chances of receiving a damaged chromosome inherited from a common ancestor. Inbreeding increases the probability of a child being born with a double dosage of one or more recessive genetic problems that congenital disabilities can cause. Inbreeding is the production of offspring from the mating or breeding of individuals or organisms that are genetically related (Jiménez, 1994). By analogy, the term is used in human reproduction. However, it more commonly refers to the genetic disorders and other consequences that may arise from the expression of deleterious or recessive traits resulting from incestuous sexual relationships and consanguinity. Inbreeding results in homozygosis, which can increase the chances of offspring being affected by deleterious or recessive traits (Bernstein et al. 1985). This usually leads to at least temporarily decreased biological fitness of a population, called inbreeding depression (Fareed and Afzal 2016). An individual who inherits such deleterious traits is colloquially referred to as inbred (ibid).

The avoidance of expression of such deleterious recessive alleles caused by inbreeding via- inbreeding avoidance mechanisms is the main selective reason for outcrossing. Crossbreeding between populations often positively affects fitness-related traits but sometimes leads to adverse effects known as outbreeding depression. However, increased homozygosis increases the probability of fixing beneficial alleles and decreases the likelihood of fixing deleterious alleles in a population. Inbreeding can purge deleterious alleles from a population through purifying selection (Fareed et al., 2017). Studies revealed that inbreeding may be one of the causes of autism in the offspring. For example, in Turkey, a recent public health campaign discourages cousin marriages with premarital screening and diagnosis for consanguineous couples, which represents the government's attempt to reduce the incidence of autism spectrum disorder (Finkler 2001). Similarly, the Chinese government has already restricted consanguineous marriage by laws to reduce autism spectrum disorder (ASD).

Gene Mutation through Consanguinity

A gene mutation is a permanent alteration in the DNA sequence that makes up a gene. The sequence may differ from person to person, but it is found in most people. Mutations range in size; they can affect a single DNA building block (base pair) to a large chromosome segment that includes multiple genes. Recall that the DNA sequence is found within a gene that controls protein synthesis. If the DNA sequence is altered, the amino acid sequence within a protein can be changed. Protein synthesis first creates an mRNA copy of a DNA sequence during transcription. This mRNA is translated into a sequence of amino acids by the ribosome. In this way, the information encoded in the sequence of bases in the DNA making up a gene is used to produce a protein. Gene mutations can be classified in two significant ways, viz. (1) hereditary mutation and (2) acquired or somatic mutation.

Figure 5 details the process of gene mutation. Autism-acquired or somatic gene mutations have been explained individually.

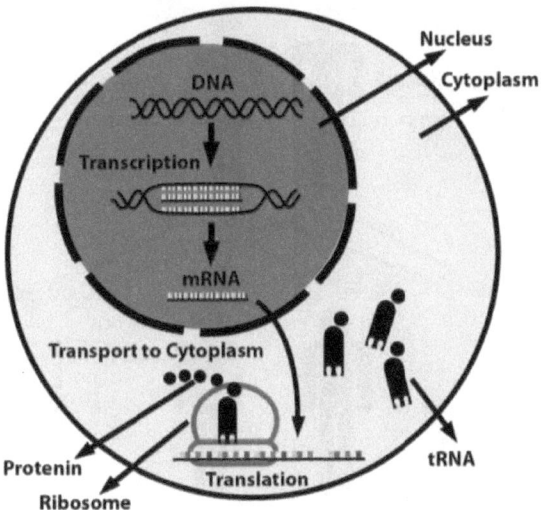

Fig. 5: Process of Gene Mutation through Consanguinity

- **Hereditary Gene Mutation (HGM):** Hereditary gene mutations are inherited from a parent and are present throughout a person's life in virtually every cell in the body. These mutations are also called germline mutations because they are present in the parent's egg or sperm cells, also called germ cells. When an egg and a sperm cell unite, the resulting fertilized egg cell receives DNA from both parents. If this DNA has a mutation, the child that grows from the fertilized egg will have the mutation in each cell.

- **Acquired Gene Mutation (SGM):** Acquired or somatic mutations occur at some time during a person's life and are present only in specific cells, not in every cell in the body. These changes can be caused by environmental factors, such as ultraviolet radiation from the sun, or can occur if a mistake is made, as DNA copies itself during cell division. Acquired mutations in somatic cells (cells other than sperm and egg cells) cannot be passed on to the next generation. In Figure 6, the white individual has inherited two mutated alleles of a gene from the parents. This is an example of a hereditary mutation. The color variation in this tulip is caused by a somatic mutation that occurred early in the development of this individual flower (Fuster and Colantonio 2004).

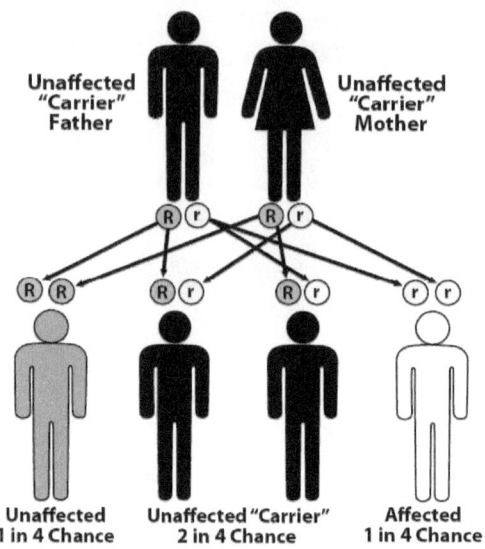

Fig. 6: Acquired GeneMutation

Genetic changes described as de novo (new) mutations can be hereditary or somatic. In some cases, the mutation occurs in a person's egg or sperm cell but is not present in any of the person's other cells. In other cases, the mutation occurs in the fertilized egg shortly after the egg and sperm cells unite. It is often impossible to tell precisely when a *de novo* mutation happened. As the fertilized egg divides, each resulting cell in the growing embryo will have a mutation. *De novo* mutations may explain genetic disorders in which an affected child has a mutation in every cell in the body. However, the parents do not, and there is no family history of the disorder.

Somatic mutations in a single cell early in embryonic development can lead to a situation called mosaicism. These genetic changes are not present in a parent's egg or sperm cells or the fertilized egg but happen later when the embryo includes several cells. As all the cells divide during growth and development, cells that arise from the cell with the altered gene will mutate, while others will not. Depending on the mutation and how many cells are affected, mosaicism may or may not cause health problems.

Most disease-causing gene mutations are uncommon in the general population. However, other genetic changes occur more frequently.

Genetic alterations in more than 1 percent of the population are called polymorphisms. They are familiar enough to be considered a normal variation in the DNA. Polymorphisms are responsible for many of the average differences between people, such as eye color, hair color, and blood type. Although many polymorphisms have no adverse effects on a person's health, some variations may influence the risk of developing certain disorders.

Impact on Consanguinity

Genetic disorders are one of the significant childhood health problems that take place due to the consanguineous marriages of the parents. Treatment and rehabilitation of children with genetic disorders is costly, and complete recovery is usually impossible. Genetic disorders are far more common than is widely appreciated and represent only the tip of the iceberg (Grant and Bittles 1997). Consanguineous marriage increases the risk of mutated autosomal recessive gene (ARG) expression and consequently increases the risk of inheriting genetic disorders among the offspring. The probability of inheriting genetic disorders depends on the closeness of the relationship between the spouses as husband and wife. That is why considerable attention has been attracted to consanguineous marriage as a causative factor of genetic disorders. It was found that the rate of consanguinity is very high among the Muslim countries. Minimal data regarding the rate of consanguinity and the prevalence of genetic disorders related to consanguinity are available in Bangladesh.

It is found in this research that the parents who are involved in cousin marriages have a high rate of their children being affected by autism compared to the parents who have non-consanguineous marital backgrounds. Consanguinity is always harmful for genetic disorders of the offspring whose parents are involved in blood-related marriage. Under the circumstances, it is necessary to introduce an awareness program to avoid consanguineous marriages to protect future generations from genetic disorders.

Concluding Remarks

Bangladesh has many achievements in the health sector. However, sufficient initiatives have yet to be taken to control genetic disorders by informing, motivating, and discouraging people about consanguineous marriage. Because consanguinity is always harmful for genetic disorders of the offspring whose parents are involved in blood-related marriage, under these circumstances, it is necessary to introduce awareness programs to avoid consanguineous marriages and protect future generations from genetic disorders. The coming generation should make them assets as the nation's human resources instead of liabilities.

References

American Psychiatric Association. (2013). *Diagnostic and Statistical Manual of Mental Disorders.* Arlington: American Psychiatric Publishing Ltd.

Anderson, N. F. (1986). "Cousin Marriage in Victorian England," *Journal of Family History,* 11(3): 285–301.

Begum, R., and F. Mamin. (2019). "Impact of Autism Spectrum Disorder on Family." *Autism-Open Access,* 9(4):34–44.

Bernstein, H., H. C. Byerly, F. A. Hopf, and R. E. Michod. (1985). "Genetic Damage, Mutation, and the Evolution of Sex." *Science.* 229 (4719): 1277–81.

Bittles, A. H. (2012). *Consanguinity in Context.* Cambridge: Cambridge University Press.

Fareed, M., and M. Afzal. (2014). "Evidence of Inbreeding Depression on Height, Weight, and Body Mass Index: A Population-Based Child Cohort Study." *American Journal of Human Biology.* 26 (6): 784–95.

———. (2016). "Increased Cardiovascular Risks associated with Familial Inbreeding: a Population-Based Study of Adolescent Cohort." *Annals of Epidemiology.* 26 (4): 283–92.

Fareed. M., Ahmad M. Kaisar, Anwar M. Azeem, and M. Afzal. (2017). "Impact of Consanguineous Marriages and Degrees of Inbreeding on Fertility, Child Mortality, Secondary Sex Ratio, Selection Intensity, and Genetic Load: A Cross-Sectional Study from Northern India." *Pediatric Research,* 81 (1): 18–26.

Finkler, K. (2001). "The Kin in the Gene: the Medicalization of Family and Kinship in American Society." *Current Anthropology,* 42(3): 235–263.

Fuster, V., and S. E. Colantonio. (2004). "Socioeconomic, Demographic, and Geographic Variables Affecting the Diverse Degree of Consanguineous Marriage in Spain." *Human Biology*, (76): 1–14.

Grant, J. C., and A. H. Bittles. (1997). "The Comparative Role of Consanguinity in Infant and Childhood Mortality in Pakistan." *Annals in Human Genetics*, 61(1):143–9.

Jiménez, J. A., K. A. Hughes, G. Alaks, L. Graham, and R. C. Lacy. (1994). "An Experimental Study of Inbreeding Depression in a Natural Habitat." *Science*, 266 (5183): 271–3.

Kelly, J. A. (1983). *Treating Child Abusive Families: Intervention based on Skills Training Principles*. New York: Plenum Press.

Modell, B., and A. Darr. (2002). "Science and Society: Genetic Counseling and Customary Consanguineous Marriage." *National Reviews Genetics*, 12 (3):225–229.

Sarker, Profulla C. (2015). "Consanguinity, Inbreeding and their Impact on Reproductive Health and Human Development in Inbred Communities." *The Indian Journal of Anthropology*, 3 (2): 69–80.

Chapter 7

PERCEPTIONS, BELIEFS, AND MYTHS ABOUT AUTISM SPECTRUM DISORDER

Introduction

There are many misconceptions associated with individuals with autism spectrum disorder (ASD). There is no known single cause of ASD. Since no two individuals with autism are the same, it is imperative to consider autism as a spectrum. This means that symptoms can appear vastly different from one person to another. For example, there are people with autism who are not verbal, or they do not communicate vocally with spoken words, while others may be verbal and very expressive with the use of words or vocal language. How autistic traits are displayed in any individual varies widely from person to person. Research clarifies some common myths about autism spectrum disorder (ASD) and offers resources for further information. The service providers, physicians, educators, the larger community, those on the spectrum, and those who care for these individuals can benefit from learning more about what is and is not true about autism. Under the circumstances, the researchers have already explored some of the standard pattern perceptions of the parents about ASD in their offspring.

Parents' Perception of ASD

The study has explored parents' perceptions of autism spectrum disorder (ASD), but the findings of this study are difficult to generalize because unrepresentative and small samples limit this study. Moreover, methods used to collect parent etiological perceptions about ASD are inconsistent and rarely comprehensive. One study has examined parental beliefs about the cause of their child's ASD using a large sample of parents and found that 40 percent attributed the cause to genetics and 41.6 percent to an external attribute (e.g., vaccinations). Most families believed there to be a multifaceted explanation for their child's ASD. Another study that sought to understand parental perceptions about ASD found that parents perceived more than one cause of ASD, with genetics, vaccinations, and environmental factors being the most frequently endorsed beliefs. Autism spectrum disorder (ASD) is associated with higher levels of anxiety for parents (Dunn et al. 2001). Providing medical information about autism etiology is the first step to helping parents to understand their child's disorder and to cope with it. The medical community accepts that autism is a neurodevelopmental disorder in which genes play a vital role but that environmental factors likely contribute as well (Inglese and Elder 2009). This conception can meet parent's beliefs constructed on their cultural values and personal experiences. In line with causal attribution theory, it is essential to consider parental perception because it can impact the treatment choices and the child's developmental trajectory (Hebert and Koulouglioti 2015). It has been reported that vaccine hesitancy may be more common among parents of children with autism spectrum disorders.

It was found in the literature review that parents hold a wide variety of perceptions about the cause of their child's autism, including genetic factors, events surrounding the child's birth, and environmental influences in the early childhood period. Some parents continue to attribute their child's autism to immunizations, although more recent studies suggest the frequency may be decreasing. Some parents are pessimistic about their child's future, while others are hopeful that new strategies will be developed. Some parents trust that society will accept their child's idiosyncrasies more. Parents' perceptions about the cause of their child's autism have been found to have an impact on decisions regarding future health care, family planning, and maternal mental health. The link between parental perceptions and their intervention choices has yet to be empirically explored.

Beliefs in the Etiology of ASD

Beliefs associated with the etiology of autism and the psychosocial adjustment of the parents with their autistic children in unavoidable situations. It is believed that the etiology of autism is an instinct in the mindset of the parents, especially the mothers, due to fate, karma, and supernatural spirits (Kirkpatrick 1979). Some of the parents of autistic children attributed that the autism of their children is associated with fate. They expressed that what happened to their children was already written on their foreheads. It is also believed that karma is the cosmic system of reward and punishment according to one's deeds in the past lives (Sarker 2017). Some of the parents thought that one of the causes of autism in their children was a sin committed by them or their forefathers in the past.

In many cultures, the etiology of autism depends upon the unseen forces or supernatural powers that intervene in human affairs. It is believed that if anyone offends them, the mystical powers punish by sickness, death, or natural calamities that destroy lives, crops, and properties. It is also believed that since human life is governed by forces of nature like sun, wind, water … and numerous supernatural forces are living around the people to control them. Under these circumstances, human life is insecure, and supernatural forces guide human beings at every step. It is believed that the wrong notions of the concerned supernatural spirits cause different types of diseases, including autism.

The usual theory of diseases is caused by the breach of some taboos or by hostile spirits or ghosts. It is a common belief that a sickness like autism is the routine punishment given by supernatural spirits if they are dissatisfied with the performance of the people. It is also believed that ancestral spirits cause similar afflictions by casting their evil eye and evil breath on human beings if they are dissatisfied with their performance. These forces are believed to have unlimited power (Sarker 2020). It is further assumed that if general people honor the spirits, they will be rewarded with good health for themselves and their children.

Myths and Facts about Autism

Autism belongs to developmental disabilities that are frequently characterized by brain-functioning complications. When a child is diagnosed with autism, it is most likely that they will need treatments and services that will help them cope with developmental and behavioral issues. The lack of understanding about autism can make it difficult for people on the autism spectrum to have their condition recognized and for them to access the support they need. False and often negative perceptions about the condition, as well as misconceptions, can lead to some people with autism being isolated and, in extreme cases, lead to abuse and bullying. There is an increasing body of research about screening for, diagnosing, and treating children with ASD. It has been reported that some of the common myths and facts associated with autism are explained here to get a clear idea.

- **Autistic Children Are *Sick*:** The common misperception about autism is that autistic children are sick, and most of the parents depend upon the Almighty God for the cure of their babies. Close family members and relatives often express a deep sense of frustration in front of autistic children, as if they are cursed with autism. There is a plethora of scientific studies that indicate many children on the spectrum feel anxious, disturbed, and exhausted when people around them are upset and express such frustrations.

    As many autistic children have a very keen sense of the emotional states of others, probably more than neurotypical people, they fall into the vicious cycle of emotional conflicts and do not know how to tackle them, leading to emotional turmoil. The universal truth is that there is no one-size-fits-all treatment for autism, and the goal of the existing clinical and nonclinical methods is to maximize children's ability to function by supporting development and learning.

- **Vaccines Cause Autism:** One of the biggest myths of all is that vaccines, specifically the MMR vaccine, cause autism. The safety of vaccinations has been repeatedly tested across large groups of people. High-quality research studies involving hundreds of thousands of people have consistently shown that vaccinations do not cause autism. There is evidence that both genetics and environment play a role in autism spectrum disorder (ASD). However, the cause of autism is not clear. Researchers have identified genes associated with autism in some populations. They also hypothesized that genes could become expressed in a person's behavior based on experiences they have throughout life. This, by no means, suggests that parents are at fault for their child's autism.

Researchers have also found a difference between the development of several areas of the brain in people who have autism spectrum disorder and those who do not, which gives more support for genes being a factor in one having autism. Additionally, children born prematurely are at a higher risk of having autism than children born full-term. A wide range of environmental factors may also influence how genes are expressed. The idea that parental practices are to blame for autistic children has been discredited. Parents do not cause their children to have autism. Also, research has indicated that children who receive vaccines are no more likely than children who do not receive vaccines to have autism spectrum disorder (Davidson 2017).

- **Environmental Risk Factors:** Studies revealed that the environmental risk factors associated with ASD include (1) advanced paternal age which is over thirty-four years, (2) poor maternal physical and mental health, (3) maternal prenatal medication use, (4) maternal exposure to chemicals, (5) preterm birth, (6) complications during birth, (7) low birth weight, (8) jaundice, and (9) post birth infections (Karimi et al. 2016). Mumps, measles, and rubella are among the infections associated with an increased risk of ASD, so the preventative MMR vaccine helps mitigate the risk of developing ASD from these infections.

- **Everyone with Autism:** Everyone with autism is unique and valuable in their own way. Autism is a *spectrum* disorder, which means that every person with autism experiences things in their way. Myths like the above add to the misconceptions about autism and early intervention. As parents, embracing their child's uniqueness and providing early support is the best they can do. Autism is not curable, but with the right tools, many on the spectrum can lead successful lives.

- **Autism in a Childhood Condition:** Autism is not a childhood condition; instead, it is a lifelong problem, and there are more autistic adults than children. Autistic adults have been overlooked in research, though many organizations are supporting several studies to find the best ways to help them at every stage of their lives. Research suggests that outcomes can change for people over time if they get the proper support, such as language, communication, and anxiety (Bishop 2007).

- **Autistic Children Are *Talented*:** The second most common misconception among many about autism is that autistic children are extraordinarily talented and exhibit phenomenal mental abilities. People try to assure their parents by bestowing comfort that autistic children have the potential and aspirations to become astronauts in NASA or the next generation of Elon Musk. Though they are not less intelligent than other children, such misconceptions create social overload and push the child into a panic.

  Research has revealed that children with ASD have greater degrees of stress chemicals in their nervous system because the system usually remains taxed and drained throughout the day. Even most of the daily school tasks drain away their energy. Therefore, loftier intellectual expectations from children on the spectrum build up the stress chemicals quickly, and by the time autistic children realize it, their coping skills often collapse.

  The paramount truth is that children with autism may or may not be aberrantly intelligent, just like others in society. It is essential to realize that every autistic kid has their own pace of doing things, and we must respect their emotional states and intelligence by neither overstating nor undermining them.

- **Autistic Children Are *Abnormal*:** Whenever the parents attempt to tell the truth by introducing their child as an autistic child, they receive an overwhelmingly bizarre reaction from many. Some people even get enraged at them for the word *autistic* the parents use. It is common in our culture that people often wonder if they should say "person with autism" or "autistic person" when talking about children or adults on the spectrum.

Autistic is not an offensive term. However, it is better to apply a person-first style when introducing someone with autism. The way we introduce a person with autism reflects how we think about it and how we prioritize their needs. Though there is no globally accepted uniform approach to addressing the issue, calling a person with autism "autistic" needs to be recognized, affirmed, and validated individual identity as an autistic person and never treated as a tragedy or curse for the family. Instead of coming to a concrete way of introducing a person with autism, it is firmly believed in individual freedom to identify a person with autism in the decent way possible within the globally accepted appropriate terms.

- **Autistic Children Are *Mad* and *Violent*:** It has been observed that many people speculate and hypothesize that autistic children are violent and that they remain extraordinarily vigilant when children with autism visit them in their places. Sometimes, people in contrasting situations try to forge extra comfort for autistic children, which makes their behavior incompatible with neurodivergent children when they are with other neurotypical children. Such animosities make it difficult for many children on the spectrum who find emotional and behavioral regulation challenging. Since emotional and behavioral regulation are interlinked, it is a matter of basic understanding that emotional dysregulation overwhelms autistic children, and meltdowns occur quickly.

Hence, without addressing the behavior toward autistic children, it cannot be generally expected that neurodivergent children would be able to regulate their emotions, leading to behavioral dysregulations. Neurodivergent children predominantly have a poor ability to check impulses, impaired ability to assess what is needed, inability to act organized, and inability to evaluate their actions and their consequences. While reading books on parenting for children with autism, I came across pacing as an emotional and behavioral regulation technique. The technique asserts that the parent or the people around the children with autism do specific tasks with them, right alongside them, setting the pace and teaching them to match it.

In this process, they learn to pace themselves by referencing or following the person facilitating the tasks. Many people often tag the word *mad* for autistic children. Many children on the spectrum usually exhibit inappropriate behavior as defined by neurotypical people in a situation where others do not expect it. This does not necessarily mean these children cannot identify the situation's emotions or sensitivity. Many on the spectrum can feel it but cannot process it due to poor connectivity between the components in their brains. Psychologists term it the weak connectivity model of autism.

We all are probably aware that the right side of the human brain deals with emotional, intuitive, and subjective reasoning. In contrast, the left side is the brain's more factual, logical, and intellectual thinking part. Identifying, labeling, evaluating, understanding, and controlling emotional sensitivity exclusively depends on integrating our right and left brains. With many on the spectrum, the brain's logical part cannot adequately interpret poor left-right brain integration, so emotional sensitivity. Scientific studies indicate a deficiency in left-right brain integration that leads to lowered emotional sensitivity due to a lack of interpretation by the logical part of the brain.

- **Cognitive Disabilities and Cannot Speak:** It is not appropriate to say that all autistic individuals are incapable of communicating or to assume that all people with autism also have an intellectual or cognitive disability. Even though cognitive or intellectual disabilities or speech disorders can co-occur with autism spectrum disorder, this does not mean that all people with autism experience these things. Many people with autism speak and communicate

Perceptions, Beliefs, and Myths about Autism Spectrum Disorder

verbally, whereas other people with autism may not be able to do so.

People with autism spectrum disorder (ASD) have some social and communication differences compared to the general population. However, autism is a spectrum, which means that every person will experience social and communication differences in their way. Some may be able to speak with words, while others may not. Instead, they may learn to communicate with gestures, body language, picture exchange systems, sign language, or electronic means.

- **Autistic People Have Learning Difficulties:** With the proper support and a suitable environment, many autistic people are very able and independent. Studies revealed that around 1 in 4 autistic people speak few or no words but can find other ways to communicate through symbolic interaction. Some autistic people take longer to process information, but it does not mean they do not understand. Autistic people also have strengths over those without autism. For example, strong attention to detail and a unique ability to see data patterns can bring many advantages.

- **Autistic People Are Anti-Social:** Autistic people may need support with social skills or interact differently with the world around them, but most autistic people enjoy having relationships. People show their social difficulties in different ways. Some are quiet and shy or avoid social situations; others speak too much and struggle to have two-way conversations. Unspoken communication can be confusing for autistic people, but body language, tone of voice, and sarcasm can be complex for them to read. These challenges can make making friends, building relationships, or getting on at work difficult. Taking time to get to know autistic people and understand their differences in an environment where they are happy makes all the difference.

- **Social Interaction Is Impaired:** Although social interaction is impaired in people with ASD, this does not mean that they cannot form relationships with others. Individuals with ASD can and do have fulfilling relationships with family, friends, spouses, and children. In contrast to the previously dominant idea that they prefer social isolation, recent studies have demonstrated that most people with ASD want to form relationships with others (Brownlow et al. 2015). Personal testimonies by individuals on the spectrum support this finding. Despite such desire, it is still difficult for people with ASD to navigate social relationships and understand social cues. Social media and other forms of online networking can help those with ASD form and maintain relationships with others both on and off the spectrum. In addition, those without ASD need to understand the perspective of their friends on the spectrum. Individuals with ASD, for instance, might be blunt and will not sugarcoat their thoughts in a way that is expected in typical social situations, which can offend others. As long as individuals without ASD are sensitive to such differences, genuine and long-lasting social relationships are possible between individuals with and without ASD (Blaxton and Bergeman 2017).

- **Create Classroom Environments:** Teachers should create classroom environments that support students with ASD in forming social relationships with their classmates. Students with ASD benefit from frequent opportunities to interact with their peers with and without ASD in inclusive environments. In addition, teachers can explicitly educate other students on how to form and maintain friendships with their classmates on the spectrum.

- **Autistic Child Does Not Feel Emotions:** There is no truth to the idea that people with autism do not have emotions or even that they cannot care about other people's emotions. People with autism experience all types of emotions. Sometimes, people with autism may have trouble interpreting others' emotions and body language or understanding social cues. They might prioritize their feelings over others. However, that is not strictly "an autism thing" since many people can do this. On the other hand, some people with autism are more observant and considerate than the average person. These people can sense others' emotions very well. They might even be considered people-pleasers because they are incredibly considerate of others, focus on other people's wants and needs more than their own, and are very sensitive to other people's experiences.

- **Autism Is a Lifelong Condition**: While autism is different for everyone, most autistic adults and families that they speak to feel that autism is a big part of their life and not something that they would take away. The objective of much research is to provide support and services to autistic people so that they need to live a long, healthy, and happy life. Autism is a complex condition that affects everyone differently, so the studies focus the efforts on the questions that autistic people tell us they want answered. Autism is a lifelong condition. Appropriate therapy and intervention can help address specific concerns, help the person develop new skills, help improve communication and social abilities, and improve the overall quality of life for people with autism.

- **Only Boys Are Autistic:** Studies revealed that in most cases, autism appears to be more common in boys. However, girls are more likely to mask their autism, learning the skills to interact with the world better than boys. Autism is also more commonly diagnosed in males, especially males during their childhood, as compared to females. However, more and more is being learned about autism in females. Although sometimes autism is thought of as only being something experienced by boys, it is also experienced by girls. This can mean that many autistic girls get a diagnosis much later in life than boys because of gender discrimination, especially where the society is patriarchal.

- **One Can Outgrow Autism:** Some people think that people with autism spectrum disorder can outgrow autism. It is true that sometimes, a child who receives intensive and effective services to address their challenges related to ASD may experience improvements in their functioning and eventually have fewer challenges that interfere with their daily life. They might even live a completely independent life that looks much like many other people's lives. However, even in these situations, the person is still likely to have autism, even if their symptoms are hard to detect. For instance, they may find having small talk difficult, get overwhelmed being around people for an extended period, or they might continue having stereotypical behaviors throughout adulthood.

- **Autism Is Caused by Bad Parenting:** Autism is not caused by bad parenting. Research has proved that parenting is not to blame because autism is a genetic disorder. Under the circumstances, many organizations support parents and help them better understand autism. This approach can improve an autistic child's communication skills. Parenting style can certainly help an autistic child cope with the world, but it is not the root cause of autistic behavior (Benson 2010).

- **Autism Is Caused by Bad Environment:** There is evidence that both genetics and environment play a role in autism spectrum disorders. However, the cause of autism is not clear. Researchers have identified genes associated with autism in some populations. They also hypothesize that genes can become expressed in a person's behavior based on experiences throughout life. This by no means suggests that parents are at fault for their child's autism.

Researchers have also found a difference between the development of several areas of the brain in people who have autism spectrum disorder and those who do not, which gives more support for genes being a factor in one having autism. Additionally, children born prematurely are at a higher risk of having autism than children born full-term. A wide range of environmental factors may also influence how genes are expressed. The idea that parental practices are to blame for autistic children has been discredited. Parents do not cause their children to have autism. Also, research has indicated that children who receive vaccines are no more likely than children who do not receive vaccines to have autism spectrum disorder (Al Anbar et al. 2010).

- **Autism Is Either Nonverbal or a Savant:** ASD is a neurodevelopment disorder that occurs on a spectrum. ASD is characterized by (1) deficits in social communication and interaction across contexts and (2) restricted and repetitive patterns of behavior, interests, or activities (American Psychiatric Association, 2013). These impairments, however, vary widely in terms of severity, impact on daily living, and effects on classroom performance. Language deficits, for instance, can range from impaired social communication to poor comprehension to a lack of speech. Some adults with ASD can live independently, while others require a great deal of support. The diagnosis of ASD covers a broad range of functions and includes the former diagnoses of Asperger's disorder, childhood disintegrative disorder, and pervasive developmental disorder.

- **People with Autism Do Have Savant Skills:** Theory enhancing this myth, which depicts all autistic people as savants, this myth has become more prevalent. People with actual savant syndrome exhibit extraordinary and exceptional abilities typically based on having a higher-than-average skill in a particular area. For example, memory, music, art, or outstanding math skills. However, less than 1 in 10 or 10 percent of individuals with autism display some advanced level of a specific skill. Among those who have a savant skill, the skills themselves vary.

  Autism sometimes involves becoming very obsessed or intensely interested in one specific topic. This fixated interest becomes so intense that the person spends excessive time and energy on the topic. Thus, they might know more about the subject than the average person. Understandably, this might lead to confusion over whether these children have savant-like abilities.

- **Autistic People Are Suitable for Jobs:** Since autism is a spectrum disorder (ASD), there is no specific type of job that will be appropriate for all individuals with ASD. While many adults with ASD may enjoy repetitive tasks, it is incorrect to assume a job is a good match solely based on a disability label. Individuals with ASD have many diverse strengths, talents, and skills that would benefit employers. Unfortunately, the unemployment rate is estimated to be between 50 and 75 percent for adults with ASD, and many of those who do have jobs are underemployed (Hendricks 2010). One reason for this is that individuals with ASD often lack the social skills necessary to be successful during job interviews and in the workplace. Specialisterne is an organization devoted to helping individuals with ASD find and maintain employment. They match employees with ASD with a coach who guides them through the social situations encountered at work. Ultimately, it is essential to consider the strengths, needs, interests, and preferences of the person with autistic spectrum disorders (ASD) pursuing employment.

This has important implications for teachers working with students with ASD. Students should have an opportunity to explore various career paths throughout their school years, and educators should not limit students' options simply because they have ASD. Transition plans should be created with the student's skills and interests in mind. In addition, teachers should not rule out college opportunities for their students with ASD. Teachers have a responsibility to help students develop skills that will enable them to be successful in their chosen post-secondary education and career path.

- **Autism Can Be Cured:** There is evidence that autism spectrum disorders can not be cured. However, early and intensive behavioral treatment can, in many cases, reduce the severity of symptoms and help individuals develop adaptive skills for daily living, emotion and behavior regulation, and social engagement.

- **Autistic Children Have No Sense of Humor:** This may be true for some people with autism, but the individual is likelier to express or share humor in unique or less obvious ways. Many parents report that their family members may tease, tell jokes, or mimic comedy actions or lines appropriately, anticipating others to be entertained.

- **Individuals with Autism Are Violent:** Though there has been recent information relating autism to violence, aggressive acts from autistic individuals usually arise from sensory overload or emotional distress, and it is unusual for individuals with autism to act violently out of malice or pose any danger to society. Many individuals prefer to limit their exposure and interactions with other people because social situations can feel confusing and anxiety-provoking.

Concluding Remarks

Autism is one of the most common mental problems faced by children across the world. There are some common perceptions, beliefs, myths, and facts about the etiology of autism, which are constantly increasing. It is necessary to combine the efforts of parents, healthcare specialists, and educators to reach the best outcomes. Out of the variety of treatment approaches, parents select those which they consider the most reliable or suitable for their child. It is crucial to provide support to children who have autism to make their assimilation into society easier. Although the exact cause of ASD remains unclear, research on ASD etiology has suggested two main contributing factors: genetics and the environment. There are also possible interactions between genes and the environment, suggesting that ASD could be a multifactorial disorder of the two factors; genetics play a more significant and critical role than environmental factors.

References

Al Anbar, N. Nebal, R. M. Dardennes, A. Prado-Netto, K. Kaye, and Y. Contejean. (2010). "Treatment Choices in Autism Spectrum Disorder: The Role of Parental Illness Perceptions." *Research in Developmental Disabilities*, 31(3):817–28.

American Psychiatric Association. (2013). *Diagnostic and Statistical Manual of Mental Disorders.* Washington: APA Publications.

Bauman, M. L. (2010)." Medical Comorbidities in Autism: Challenges to Diagnosis and Treatment." *Neurotherapeutics*, 7(4): 320–327.

Benson, Paul R. (2010). "Coping, Distress, and Well-being in Mothers of Children with Autism." *Research in Autism Spectrum Disorders*, 4(2):217–28.

Bishop, S. L., J. Richler, A. C. Cain, and C. Lord. (2007). "Predictors of Perceived Negative Impact in Mothers of Children with Autism Spectrum Disorder." *American Journal on Mental Retardation*, 112(6):450–61.

Blaxton, J. M., and C. S. Bergeman. (2017). "A Process-Oriented Perspective Examining the Relationships among Daily Coping, Stress, and Affect." Personality and Individual Differences, 104(1):357–61.

Bölte, S.; S. Girdler, and P. B. Marschik. (2019). "The Contribution of Environmental Exposure to the Etiology of Autism Spectrum Disorder." Life Science, 76 (4): 1275–1297.

Boterberg, S., T. Charman, P. B. Marschik, S. Bolte, and H. Roeyers. (2019). "Regression in Autism Spectrum Disorder: A Critical Overview of Retrospective Findings and Recommendations for Future Research." *Neuroscience Biobehavioral Review*, 102 (1): 24–55.

Brownlow, C., H. B. Rosqvist, and L. O'Dell. (2015). "Exploring the Potential for Social Networking among People with Autism:

Challenging Dominant Ideas of 'Friendship.'" *Scandinavian Journal of Disability Research,* 17(2): 188–193.

Davidson, M. (2017). "Vaccination as a Cause of Autism-myths and Controversies." Dialogues in Clinical Neuroscience, 19(4): 403–407

Dunn, M. E., T. Burbine, C. A. Bowers, and S. Tantleff-Dunn. (2001). "Moderators of Stress in Parents of Children with Autism." *Commune Mental Health Journal,* 3(1): 39–52.

Geschwind, D. H. (2011). Genetics of Autism Spectrum Disorders. *Trends Cognitive Science,* 15(4): 409–416.

Goin-Kochel, R. P., S. S. Mire, and A. G. Dempsey. (2015). "Emergence of Autism Spectrum Disorder in Children from Simplex Families: Relations to Parental Perceptions of Etiology." Journal of Autism Development Disorder, 45 (3): 1451–1463.

Hebert, E. B., and C. Koulouglioti. (2015). "Parental Beliefs about Cause and Course of Their Child's Autism and Outcomes of their Beliefs: A Review of the Literature." *Journal of Pediatrics Nursing,* 28 (3): 149–163.

Hendricks, D. (2010). "Employment and Adults with Autism Spectrum Disorders: Challenges and Strategies for Success." *Journal of Vocational Rehabilitation,* 32(2): 125-134

Inglese, M. D., and J. H. Elder. (2009). "Caring for Children with Autism Spectrum Disorder." *Journal of Pediatrics Nursing,* 24 (2): 41-48.

Karimi, P., E. Kamali, S. M. Mousavi, and M. Karahmadi. (2016). "Environmental Factors Influencing the Risk of Autism." *Journal of Research in Medical Sciences,* 21(11): 1–12.

Kirkpatrick Joanna. (1979). *The Sociology of an Indian Hospital.* Calcutta: Firma KLM Private Limited.

Lintas, C., A. M. and Persico. (2009). "Autistic Phenotypes and Genetic Testing: State-of-the-Art for the Clinical Geneticist." *Journal of Medical Genetics*, 9(1): 1–8.

Robert, C., L. Pasquier, D. Cohen, M. Fradin, R. Canitano, L. Damaj, and S. Tordjman. (2017). "Role of Genetics in the Etiology of Autistic Spectrum Disorder: Toward a Hierarchical Diagnostic Strategy." *International Journal of Molecular Science*, 18 (3): 618-625.

Sarker, Profulla C. (2017). *Sociocultural Parameters of Health and Diseases*. Dhaka: Mother's Publications.

―――. (2020). *Revitalization of Traditional Medicine in Holistic Healing System: Across-Cultural Study*. Dhaka: Center for Research, Knowledge Management, and Human Resource Development, Royal University of Dhaka.

Schaefer, G. B. (2016). "Clinical Genetic Aspects of ASD Spectrum Disorders." *International Journal of Molecular Science*, 17(2): 180–190.

Chapter 8

Diagnosis, Treatment, and Knowledge of Parents about Treatment

Introduction

Autism spectrum disorder (ASD) is a complex, highly heritable neurodevelopmental disease characterized by individuals with a combination of behavioral and cognitive impairments. These include impaired or diminished social communication skills, repetitive behaviors, and restricted sensory processing or interests (Lord et al. 2020; Bauman and Kemper 2005). Swiss psychiatrist Eugen Bleuler first coined the term autism in 1908 to describe symptoms associated with severe schizophrenia, hallucinations, and unconscious fantasy among infants. Since then, the classification, diagnosis, and meaning of autism have radically changed (Evans 2013). Between the 1940s and 1980s, ASD was described as abnormalities in language development, display of ritualistic and compulsive behaviors, and disturbance in interpersonal communication in developing relationships. In the 1970s, sensory deficits in infancy were recognized among autistic children and thus contributed to defining the features of autism spectrum disorder.

In 1980, the third edition of the American Psychiatric Association's (APA) Diagnostic and Statistical Manual of Mental Disorders (DSM-III) listed autism as a subgroup within the diagnostic category of pervasive developmental disorders (PDD) to convey the view that there is a broader spectrum of social communication deficits. The PDD contained four categories: (1) infantile autism, (2) childhood-onset pervasive developmental disorders, (3) residual autism, and (4) an atypical form of ASD. At this point, it was recognized that the symptoms resembling schizophrenia were not a component of ASD. Consequently, childhood schizophrenia was excluded, which was considered earlier as one of the components of ASD. In the 1980s, Wing (1980) placed autistic children on a continuum with other abnormal children and discussed autism in behavioral terms rather than psychosis.

Wing (1980) also proposed that autism is part of a wider group of conditions that share commonalities, including impairments of communication, imagination, and social interactions. In 1990, autism was first classified as a disability (King et al. 2014). Moving to the present day, ASD is a blanket term that distinguishes individuals using clinical specifiers and modifiers. The knowledge of pathology, etiology, and behavior of ASD continues to evolve. Nowadays, ASD is widely recognized as a somewhat common condition that, for many, but not all, requires lifelong support.

Despite recent advancements in medical science in terms of mental health, psychotherapy, and physiotherapy, there are no reliable biomarkers for ASD. Consequently, today's clinical diagnosis of ASD is based on assessing behaviors. These include psychiatric disorders such as attention deficit hyperactivity disorder (ADHD), which is considered the most common comorbidity in people with ASD, along with other conditions and diseases, including anxiety and phobias, dissociative disorders, depression, bipolar disorder, episodic mood disorders (Simonoff 2008). Physiological disorders (e.g., gastrointestinal disorders) and genetic disorders (e.g., fragile X syndrome) may also be prevalent (Doshi-Velez 2014).

Early Signs and Symptoms

Early identification and evaluation of ASD in children have become a significant public health objective due to the potential association between early intervention and improved development of children with ASD (Johnson and Myers, 2007; Rogers et al., 2019). Early presentation of ASD often occurs due to parental concerns spurred by recognizing some of the hallmarks of ASD previously outlined, which has increased due to greater awareness of ASD hallmarks among parents, relatives, especially those who were involved in kinship ties, healthcare specialists, and childcare workers (Dover and LeCouteur 2007). Some video studies suggest that it is possible to identify symptoms of ASD in children as young as 6–12 months old (Baranek 2999). There is increased interest in monitoring the emergence of ASD prodromes, such as reduced motor control or abnormal social development in the first year of life (Yirmiya and Charman 2010). As research has developed, it is now known that the prevalence of ASD is exceptionally high in preterm infants, indicating a requirement for additional vigilance in preterm pregnancy.

Diagnosis of Autistic Children

Autism spectrum disorder (ASD), also known as pervasive developmental disorders (PDDs), causes severe and pervasive impairment in thinking, feeling, language, and the ability to relate or communicate to others. These disorders are usually first diagnosed in early childhood and range from a severe form, called autistic disorder, through pervasive development disorder not otherwise specified, to a much milder form, Asperger's syndrome. They also include two rare disorders, Rett syndrome and childhood disintegrative disorder. Although there are many concerns about labeling a young child with an autism spectrum disorder, the earlier the diagnosis of ASD is made, the earlier needed interventions can begin. Evidence over the last fifteen years indicates that intensive early intervention in optimal educational settings for at least two years during the preschool year results in improved outcomes in most young children with ASD. In evaluating a child, clinicians rely on behavioral characteristics to diagnose. Some of the characteristic behaviors of ASD may be apparent in the first few months of a child's life, or they may appear at any time during the early years. For the diagnosis, problems in at least one of the areas of communication, socialization, or restricted behavior must be present before age 3. The diagnosis requires a two-stage process. The first stage involves developmental screening during well-child checkups; the second stage entails a comprehensive evaluation by a multidisciplinary team.

Developmental Screening

Developmental screening is the first stage of the diagnosis of ASD. A healthy child checkup should include a developmental screening test. If a child's pediatrician does not routinely check the child with such a test, ask that it be done. Own observations of the parents and concerns about their child's development will be essential in helping to screen the child. Reviewing family videotapes, photos, and baby albums can help parents remember when each behavior was first noticed and when the child reached certain developmental milestones. Some screening instruments rely solely on parent responses to a questionnaire; some rely on parent reports and observations. Essential items on these instruments that appear to differentiate children with autism from other groups before age two include pointing and pretend play. Screening instruments do not provide individual diagnosis but serve to assess the need for referral for possible diagnosis of ASD. These screening methods may not identify children with mild ASD, such as those with high-functioning autism.

Comprehensive Diagnostic Evaluation

The second stage of diagnosis must be comprehensive to accurately rule in or rule out an ASD or other developmental problem. This evaluation may be done by a multidisciplinary team that includes a psychologist, a neurologist, a psychiatrist, a speech therapist, or other professionals like clinical social workers who diagnose children with ASD. Customarily, an expert diagnostic team is responsible for thoroughly evaluating the child, assessing the child's strengths and weaknesses, and determining a formal diagnosis. The team will then meet with the parents to explain the evaluation results. Although parents may have been aware that something was not quite right with their child, when the diagnosis is given, it is a devastating blow. At such a time, staying focused on asking questions is hard. However, while members of the evaluation team are together, the best opportunity for parents to ask questions and get recommendations on what further steps they should take for their children. Learning as much as possible at this meeting is very important, but it is helpful to leave this meeting with the name or names of professionals who can be contacted if the parents have further questions.

Diagnosis, Treatment, and Knowledge of Parents about Treatment

Diagnostic Features of ASD

The diagnostic features historically associated with ASD are a triad of impaired social interactions, verbal and nonverbal communication deficits, and restricted, repetitive behavior patterns. These core features are observed irrespective of race, ethnicity, religion, culture, or socioeconomic status. However, ASD individuals tend to differ from one another, so one feature may be more prevalent than another (Khan, 2012). The child's physician will look for signs of developmental delays at regular checkups. Suppose the child shows any symptoms of autism spectrum disorder. In that case, the parents will likely be referred to a specialist who treats children with autism spectrum disorder, such as a child psychiatrist or psychologist, pediatric neurologist, or developmental pediatrician, for an evaluation. Because autism spectrum disorder varies widely in symptoms and severity, making a diagnosis may be difficult. There is no specific medical test to determine the disorder. Instead, a specialist may observe the following diagnosis-specific features:

- Observe the child and ask how the child's social interactions, communication skills, and behavior have developed and changed over time.
- Conduct tests on the child's hearing, speech, language, developmental level, and social and behavioral issues.
- Present structured social and communication interactions to the child and score the performance.
- Use the criteria in the Diagnostic and Statistical Manual (DSM) of Mental Disorders published by the American Psychiatric Association.
- Include other specialists in determining a diagnosis.
- Recommend genetic testing to identify whether the child has a genetic disorder such as Rett syndrome or fragile X syndrome.

Diagnostic Tools

ASD is a complex disorder and may involve other neurological or genetic problems; a comprehensive evaluation should entail neurologic and genetic assessment, along with in-depth cognitive and language testing. In addition, measures developed specifically for diagnosing autism are often used. These include the Autism Diagnosis Interview-Revised (ADI-R) and the Autism Diagnostic Observation Schedule (ADOS-G). The ADI-R is a structured interview that contains over one hundred items and is conducted with a caregiver. It consists of four main factors, viz. the child's (1) communication, (2) social interaction, (3) repetitive behaviors, and (4) age-of-onset symptoms. The ADOS-G is an observational measure used to press for socio-communicative behaviors that are often delayed, abnormal, or absent in children with ASD. Another instrument that professionals usually use is the Childhood Autism Rating Scale (CARS). It aids in evaluating the (1) child's body movements, (2) adaptation to change, (3) listening response, (4) verbal communication, and (5) relationship to people. It is suitable for use with children over two years of age. The examiner observes the child and also obtains relevant information from the parents. The child's behavior is rated on a scale based on deviation from the typical behavior of children of the same age. Two other tests that should be used to assess any child with a developmental delay are a formal audiological hearing evaluation and a lead screening. Although some hearing loss can co-occur with ASD, some children with ASD may be incorrectly thought to have such a loss. In addition, if the child has suffered from an ear infection, transient hearing loss can occur. Lead screening is essential for children who remain for an extended period in the oral-motor stage, in which they put anything and everything into their mouths. Children with an autistic disorder usually have elevated blood lead levels.

Diagnostic Guideline

Numerous diagnostic guidelines of varying quality are available (Penner et al., 2018). The essential features of ASD diagnosis include observing a child's relationship and exchange with their parents and an individual unknown to the child during unstructured and structured assessment activities and a detailed history of the Child's development. ASD diagnosis can occur at any age but most frequently occurs early in childhood. Although there is a lack of universal screening instruments, public health systems in various countries in Europe, such as Spain and Ireland, have programs in place to identify young children with ASD using M-CHAT (Modified Checklist for Autism in Toddlers) and similar tools (Blank et al. 2020). The sensitivity of these screening methods has been questioned as they fail to identify most children with ASD before their parents have already reported delayed development. Studies revealed that there may also be racial disparities in early diagnosis of black and Hispanic children versus white children, which has been reported in the United States.

Inconsistencies aside, several standardized screening tools exist to diagnose ASD at an early age, many of which focus on high-risk individuals (e.g., with a family member previously diagnosed with ASD). These include the Screening Tool for Autism in Toddlers and Young Children (STAT™), a twenty-minute observation of young children established in 2000. The longer and widely researched Autism Diagnostic Observation Schedule (ADOS™) is a forty-five-minute observation conducted by a professional or clinician to diagnose ASD from twelve months to adulthood (Blank et al. 2020). Screening tools are also suitable for research, such as the Diagnostic Instrument for Social Communication Disorders (DISCO) and the Autism Diagnostic Interview-Revised (ADI-R) in the UK. Other screening tools, such as the Social Responsiveness Scale (SRS), the Social Communication Questionnaire (SCQ), and the childhood autism rating scale (CARS), can be used to assess a child's symptoms of ASD. While many tools to screen and diagnose ASD exist, two of the leading autism diagnostic tools in use today are DSM-5 and M-CHAT (Modified Checklist for Autism in Toddlers).

Treatment Processes

There is no evidence of a cure for autism spectrum disorder (ASD), and there is no one-size-fits-all treatment. Treatment aims to maximize the child's ability to function by reducing symptoms and supporting development and learning. Early intervention during the preschool years can help the child learn critical social, communication, functional, and behavioral skills (DeSouza et al., 2019).

The range of home-based and school-based treatments and interventions for autism spectrum disorder can be overwhelming, and the child's needs may change over time. The healthcare provider can recommend options and help identify resources in the local area. If the child is diagnosed with autism spectrum disorder, talk to experts about creating a treatment strategy and build a team of professionals to meet the child's needs.

Treatment Options

A treatment option is something that anybody can choose to do in preference to one or more alternatives for their treatment. Here, treatment options are confined to the following therapies for autism spectrum disorder (ASD). The emphasis on ASD patient autonomy in health care decision-making has focused predominantly on patient rights to make an informed choice between treatment options. Meanwhile, the physician has chosen the following relevant treatment options from which autistic persons can choose.

- **Behavior and Communication Therapies:** Many programs address the social, language, and behavioral difficulties of autism spectrum disorder. Some programs focus on reducing problem behaviors and teaching new skills. Other programs focus on teaching children how to act in social situations or communicate better with others. Applied behavior analysis (ABA) can help children learn new skills and generalize these skills to multiple situations through a reward-based motivation system.

- **Educational Therapies:** Children with autism spectrum disorder often respond well to highly structured educational programs. Successful programs typically include a team of specialists and various activities to improve social skills, communication, and behavior. Preschool children who receive intensive, individualized behavioral interventions often show good progress.

- **Family Therapies:** Parents and other family members can learn how to play and interact with their children in ways that promote social interaction skills, manage problem behaviors, and teach daily living skills and communication.

- **Other Therapies:** Depending on the child's needs, speech therapy to improve communication skills, occupational therapy to teach activities of daily living, and physical therapy to improve movement and balance may be beneficial. A psychologist can recommend ways to address problem behavior.

- **Medications:** No medication can improve the core signs of autism spectrum disorder, but specific medications can help control symptoms. For example, certain medications may be prescribed if the child is hyperactive; antipsychotic drugs are sometimes used to treat severe behavioral problems, and antidepressants may be prescribed for anxiety. Keep health care providers updated on any medication or supplement the child takes. Some medicines and supplements can interact, causing dangerous side effects.

Management of Health

This section deals with other management of medical and mental health conditions of autism spectrum disorder individuals. In addition to autism spectrum disorder, children, teens and adults can also experience:

- **Medical Health Issues:** Children with autism spectrum disorder may also have medical issues, such as epilepsy, sleep disorders, limited food preferences, or stomach problems. Under these circumstances, the child's doctor must ask how to best manage these conditions together.

- **Problems with Transition to Adulthood:** Teens and young adults with autism spectrum disorder may have difficulty understanding body changes. Also, social situations become increasingly complex in adolescence, and there may be less tolerance for individual differences. Behavior problems may be challenging during the teen years.

- **Other Mental Health Disorders:** Teens and adults with autism spectrum disorder often experience other mental health disorders, such as anxiety and depression. Doctors, mental health professionals, community advocacy groups, and service organizations can offer help in this situation.

Future Planning

Children with autism spectrum disorder typically continue to learn and compensate for problems throughout life, but most of them will continue to require some level of support. Planning for the child's future opportunities, such as employment, college, living situation, independence, and the necessary support services, can make this process smoother.

Challenges to High-Functioning Autism

Most cases of ASD are diagnosed around age three when certain milestones, such as speech and social development, have not been met or have regressed. However, with HFA, research has found that most are diagnosed later in childhood, between the ages of seven and nine. While it is often thought that the greater awareness about ASD contributes to early detection, decades ago, that was not the case. At that time, the kids and adults with HFA might have just been thought of as quirky, awkward, or eccentric, but now we know so much more. The following are the four common challenges in high-functioning autism (HFA):

1. **Deficits in Social Interactions:** This can include discomfort with eye contact, lack of reciprocal conversation, and difficulty with nonverbal communication, such as understanding body language and social cues. They may also have a harder time making friends due to these challenges.

2. **Dislike of Change:** Those with HFA like predictability and routine and tend to develop repetitive habits. Consequently, they can become agitated when unexpected change happens or something interferes with their preferred pattern of behavior.

3. **Restricted Areas of Interest:** They tend to be very focused—even fixated—on specific ideas or subjects. While the narrowness of their interests can be limiting, their ability to focus on a particular topic can be extraordinary.

4. **Sensory Sensitivities:** It is not unusual for people with ASD to be sensitive to sensory input. They may find certain smells, noises, tastes, light, and touch overwhelming or uncomfortable. When exposed to them, it can be very stressful and upsetting.

Strengths in High-Functioning Autism

Despite the challenges, people with high-functioning autism often have several identifiable strengths, too. Among them are

1. **Strong Ability to Concentrate:** Those with HFA tend to develop special interests and can devote long periods to learning about them. They can stay focused so that their knowledge can be channeled into vocations that they enjoy and benefit others.

2. **Higher Intelligence:** Many people with HFA are brilliant and have a great memory, a strong vocabulary, and the ability to think visually. This helps them think outside the box and be creative problem solvers.

3. **Honest and Accepting:** They will be honest and tell you the truth. Those with HFA see through pretense. They are not judgmental, prejudiced, or manipulative and accept others as they are.

4. **Very Reliable:** They tend to have much integrity and be conscientious. People with HFA are dependable, and their uncanny focus helps them follow through with commitments and promises.

Parents' Knowledge of Treatment

The prevalence of autism is increasing in Bangladesh due to inbreeding through consanguinity or consanguineous marriages. Owing to parents being the primary caregivers in most situations, their ability to recognize the signs and symptoms of autism and respond appropriately is of paramount importance in aiming to provide the best health care to their autistic offspring. This study was conducted to ascertain the parent's knowledge and awareness of autism. About 53.3 percent of parents were rated as being unfamiliar with the treatment for their autistic children or had just heard about it. On the other hand, about 33.3 percent of parents reported a limited understanding of the treatment. About 13.4 percent of parents indicated they had practical knowledge of the treatment. A graph is given here to get an idea about the parents' understanding of the treatment of their autistic children (Graph 7).

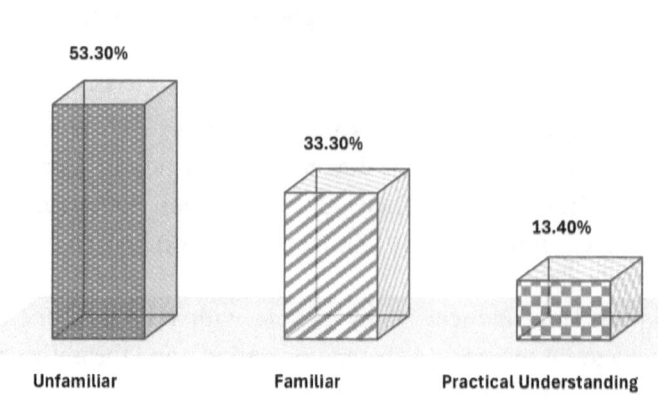

Graph 6: Level of Knowledge on Treatment

Treatment Options in the Research Area

The four treatment options parents rated themselves as most knowledgeable about are physiotherapy, occupational therapy, parent involvement, and social stories. It is not surprising that physiotherapy is well known, as it addresses core deficits in ASD. The first three treatments would be offered in special schools and hospitals, contributing to parents' knowledge. The data indicated that 78.2 percent of parents were not informed about the different treatment options before using the treatment. Families revealed that Professionals themselves are not informed about the range of ASD treatments, which could indicate a lack of professional guidance regarding which treatments to select.

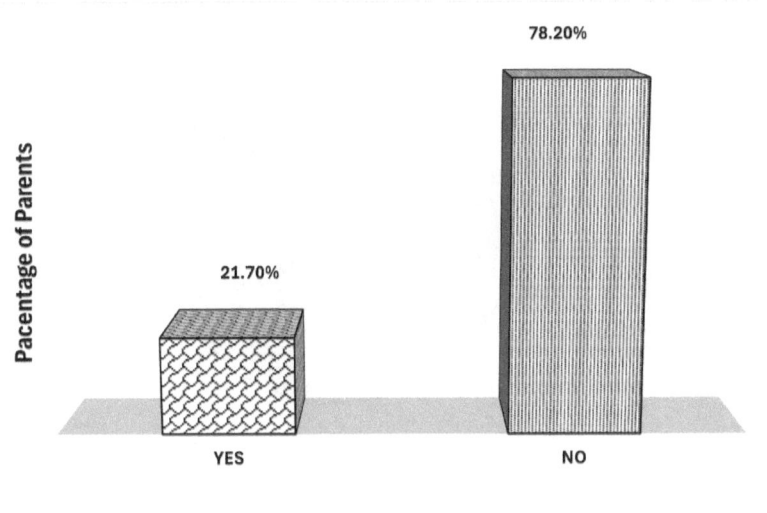

Graph 7: Parents who were informed of treatment options.

Parents' Access to Treatments

Most of the participants (i.e., 68.6 percent) stated that they had difficulty accessing treatment facilities and health professionals specializing in ASD, as depicted in Pie 3. These findings correlate that more than half of the parents (i.e., 53 percent) were unfamiliar with or had only heard of the treatments in question. In comparison, 13.4 percent had a practical understanding of the treatments. Parents rated their speech-language therapy (SLT) knowledge as the most essential treatment. On the other hand, about 68 percent of parents stated that they had difficulties accessing ASD treatment facilities and healthcare professionals and perceived treatments as being costly for the parents.

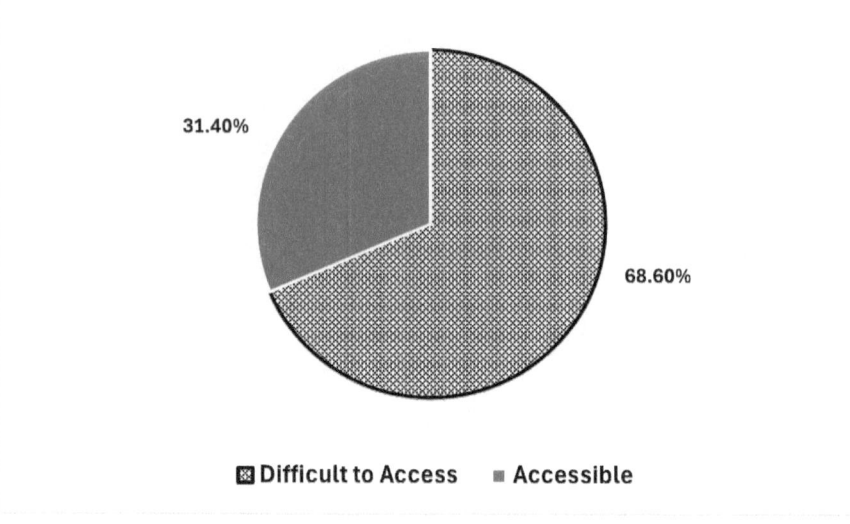

Pie 03: Parents' Access to Treatment

Challenges to Get Treatment

Challenges included limited numbers of trained health professionals and treatment facilities, long waiting lists, and long distances traveled by parents to receive treatment for their autistic children. One parent stated that 'there is no access to internet facilities yet where they would get some ideas and knowledge of a few available treatment processes. It has been reported that many of these treatments are only available in the private sector with high financial involvement. In addition, treatment facilities are concentrated in urban settings.

Concluding Remarks

If a child is diagnosed with autism spectrum disorder, first, the parents should talk to experts about creating a treatment strategy and build a team of professionals to meet the child's needs. The goal of treatment for autistic children is to maximize the child's ability to function by reducing autism spectrum disorder symptoms and supporting development and learning. Early intervention during the preschool years can help the child learn critical social, communication, functional, and behavioral skills.

Diagnosis, Treatment, and Knowledge of Parents about Treatment

The range of home-based and school-based treatments and interventions for autism spectrum disorder can be overwhelming, and the child's needs may change over time. The treatment training for parents needs to be provided full-time and lifelong by physicians to keep autistic people active. The treatment facilities for autistic children need to be expanded to rural settings with minimal cost so that everyone can avail of the treatment facilities.

References

Baranek, G. T. (2999). "Autism during Infancy: A Retrospective Video Analysis of Sensory-Motor and Social Behaviors at 9–12 Months of Age". *Journal of Autism Development Disorder,* 9(3):213–24.

Bauman, M. L. and Kemper, T. L. (2005). "Neuroanatomic Observations of the Brain in Autism: A Review and Future Directions." *International Journal of Development Neuroscience,* 23(2–3):183–187.

Blank, M. S., J. B. Turner, P. W. Fisher, E. B. Guthrie, and A. H. Whitaker. (2020). "The Need for a Clinically Useful Schema of Social Communication." *Journal of American Academy Child Adolescence Psychiatry,* 59(11):1198–200.

DeSouza, A., V. Wolan, A. Battochio, S. Christian, S. Hume, and G. Johner. (2019). "Newborn Screening: Current Status in Alberta." *Canada International Journal of Neonatal Screen,* 12 (3):5:37.

Doshi-Velez, F., Y. Ge, and I. Kohane. (2014). "Comorbidity Clusters in Autism Spectrum Disorders: An Electronic Health Record Time-series Analysis." *Pediatrics,* 133(1):e54–63.

Dover, C. J., and A. LeCouteur. (2007). "How to Diagnose Autism." Archives of Disease in Childhood, 92(6):540–545.

Evans, B. (2013). "How Autism Became Autism: The Radical Transformation of a Central Concept of Child Development in Britain." *History of Human Science,* 26(3):3–1.

Johnson, C. P., and S. M. Myers. (2007). "Identification and Evaluation of Children with Autism Spectrum Disorders." *Pediatrics,* 120(5):1183–215.

Khan, N. Z., L. A. Gallo, A. Arghir, B. Budisteanu, M. Budisteanu, I. Dobrescu, K. Donald, S. El-Tabari, M. Hoogenhout, F. Kalambayi, and R. Kawa. (2012). "Autism and the Grand Challenges in Global Mental Health". *Autism Research,* 5(3):156–159.

King, B. H., N. Navot, R. Bernier, and S. J. Webb. (2014). "Update on Diagnostic Classification in Autism". *Current Opinion Psychiatry*, 27(2):105-112.

Lord, C., T. Charman, J. Cusack, D. Guillaume, T. Frazier, R. M. Jones, P., A., L., T.J., and V. V. Jeremy. (2020). "Autism Spectrum Disorder (ASD)." *National Reviews Disease Primers*; 6(1): 34–45.

Maestro, S., F. Muratori, M. C. Cavallaro, F. Pei, D. Stern, B. Golse, and F. Palacio-Espasa. (2002). "Attentional Skills during the First Six Months of Age in Autism Spectrum Disorder." *Journal of American Acadic Child AdolescnePsychiatry,* 41(10):1239–1245.

Penner, M., E. Anagnostou, L. Y. Andoni, and W. J. Ungar. (2018). "Systematic Review of Clinical Guidance Documents for Autism Spectrum Disorder Diagnostic Assessment in Select Regions." *Autism*, 22(5):517–527.

Rogers, S. J., A. Estes, C. Lord, J. Munson, M. Rocha, J. Winter, J. Greenson, C. Colombo, G. Dawson, L. A. Vismara, and C. A. Sugar. (2019). "A Multisite Randomized Controlled Two-Phase Trial of the Early Start Denver Model Compared to Treatment as Usual." *Journal of American Academy Child Adolescence Psychiatry*, 58(9):853–865.

Simonoff, S., A. Pickles, T. Charman, S. Chandler, T. Loucas, and G. Baird. (2008). "Psychiatric Disorders in Children with Autism Spectrum Disorders: Prevalence, Comorbidity, and Associated Factors in a Population-Derived Sample." *Journal of the American Academy of Child and Adolescent Psychiatry*, 47(8):921–929.

Wing L. (1980). "Asperger's Syndrome: A Clinical Account." Psychological Medicine, 11(1):115–129.

Yirmiya, N., and T. Charman. (2010). "The Prodrome of Autism: Early Behavioral and Signs, Regression, Peri- and Post-Natal Development, and Genetics." *Journal of Child Psychology Psychiatry*, 51(4):432–58.

Chapter 9

CHALLENGES FOR PARENTS AND FAMILIES IN RAISING AUTISTIC CHILDREN

Introduction

Autism spectrum disorder (ASD) is a complex neurological disorder that affects brain function and causes impairments in multiple areas of development, including social interaction, communication, and behavior, and typically appears within the first three years of life. Parents having children with autism spectrum disorder face many challenges associated with disruptive behavior. Parents with ASD children face extreme difficulties in dealing with challenging behaviors, teaching their children to communicate, teaching basic life skills, protecting their children from danger, and preparing their children for adult life. Besides, the parents also experience high levels of stress, high recurrence risks, misconceptions and assumptions, and feelings of guilt and blame regarding the child's diagnosis. The social stigma attached to the disorder causes much discrimination not only of the autistic child but also of the parents because they are blamed as a part of the illness.

It is well recognized that caring for a child with a disability contributes to higher levels of stress than caring for a child with typical development (Dyson 1997). Caring for a child diagnosed with autism can be incredibly

Challenges for Parents and Families in Raising Autistic Children

stressful for carers (Dumas et al. 1991; Ingersoll and Hambrick 2011). As there appears to be an increasing number of children receiving a diagnosis of Autism Spectrum Disorders (Cox et al. 1999) and children are now being diagnosed much younger (Charman and Baird 2002), the continued study of factors relating to difficulties faced by the parents needs to be fully addressed. This chapter highlights the significant challenges and problems faced by parents as well as family members having children with autism.

Challenges for Parents Families

Children with autism also display repetitive, nonfunctioning activities and interests, which present considerable challenges and distress for individuals with autism as well as their families due to the individuals' intolerance of changes (Dunla et al. 1983). Routines and ritual behaviors are thought to be significantly more prevalent and marked in individuals with autism relative to age and ability-matched controls (Lord and Pickles 1996; Leekam et al. 2007). The presence of repetitive behaviors is reported as significantly stressful by parents, caregivers, and other members of families (De Meyer and Goldberg 1983; Gabriels et al. 2005; Koegel et al. 1992). The extreme distress and catastrophic reactions shown by many in response to changes in routine are rarely described in non-autistic individuals. In addition to these problems, parents also have to deal with many other co-occurring difficulties, such as the financial and time burden of medical treatment and other therapeutic interventions, restrictions on social activities, parental sense of loss and grief, and changes to family goals and achievements (McCubbin et al. 1982; Lecavalier et al. 2006). Furthermore, research suggests that there are insufficient support services for parents of children with autism, which might help them cope with stress (Whitaker 2002). Some common challenges faced by parents having children with autism are highlighted in this chapter.

- **Parental Stress:** Parents of disabled children are particularly vulnerable to stress. Studies revealed that the levels of distress are higher in mothers than fathers of severely disabled children. Studies also showed that parental distress and family functioning impact children in numerous ways, affecting their cognitive, behavioral, and social development. Although there are many other developmental disorders which present in the parents with ongoing grief, autism is unique in several ways. First, the disorder has no clear biological marker, unlike many other developmental disabilities. Second, because autism is characterized by problems of social interaction, such as forming attachments and showing affection, parents of children with autism are often denied some of the fundamental rewards of parenthood. Consequently, autism has been considered one of the most complex and intractable developmental disorders of their children with which parents may have to cope.

The common characteristics of autism that contribute to parenting stress include scattered intellectual abilities or isolated skills and pervasive problem behavior such as self-stimulatory behaviors. Other important factors associated with parental stress in families of children with autism include feelings of loss of personal control, absence of spousal support, and informal and professional support. Family members of children with autism are often perceived to experience adverse psychological effects, which may include a higher risk for depression, social isolation in kinship network relations, and marital discord.

Many parents also experience periods of disbelief, deep sadness, depression, self-blame, and guilt, whereas others experience helplessness, feelings of inadequacy, anger, shock, and shame (Gupta and Singhal, 2005). Specific stressors that contribute to parental distress include concerns over the permanency of their child's condition and poor acceptance of autistic behaviors by the community and other parents in society (Prince 2007). Mothers appear to be the most affected and experience distress and conflicting and even ambivalent emotions compared to fathers. Depression is often elevated at the time of diagnosis of a child's disability but may decline substantially over time. Chronic sorrow and a sense of failure are emotional states frequently reported by parents of autistic children (Kourkoutas et al. 2012).

- **Parenting:** Autism is a severe disability because of the intense lifelong effects it has on the individual and their family. Parents raising a child with autism face extreme difficulties in dealing with challenging behaviors, teaching their child to communicate, teaching basic life skills, guarding their child from danger, and preparing their child for adult life (Dyches et al. 2004). Kourkoutas et al. (2012) argued that there are high-risk factors that might induce acute or chronic stress and trauma in the parents of autistic children and, in turn, lead to dysfunctional parenting. The following are high-risk factors:

1. The ambiguity of diagnosis.
2. The severity and duration of the child's disorder.
3. A very low IQ.
4. Lack of congruity with the community norms, bizarre forms of communication and behavior.
5. Enduring disruptive or disorganized behaviors.

Families with autistic children have been perceived by their societies in different ways, causing the families to be shaped by the belief systems of autism specific to their society. Because of social stigma, there is much discrimination not only of the autistic child but also of the family as a whole because the family is seen to be a part of the illness. Fear of discrimination and the stigmas surrounding disabilities lead many family members to refuse to go to professionals and receive a diagnosis for their children. By refusing to be diagnosed, families can avoid having disability identities (Ecker 2010). The troublesome symptoms, such as tantrums, self-destructive acts, and other inappropriate public behaviors associated with the disorder, are challenging to cope with. Consequently, parents with autistic children frequently encounter hostile or insensitive reactions from the public, primarily because of the inappropriate behavior shown by their children.

Public reactions to such families are often stereotypical and negative (Gray 1993). Because of delayed communication in autistic children, parents may experience positive and negative changes as the children grow and enter the school system. The school system has initiated a new involvement concerning the needs of the children and the parents. It should be noted that the parents and school personnel are closely related in pursuing the most appropriate education for the child (Hoppe 2005). Caregivers of autistic children may perceive their children as having a more difficult temper mentally than other children and, therefore, use more extraordinary control strategies with their children. Thus, caregivers' perceptions of their children's characteristics may influence how they interact with their children (Kesari et al. 1997). Families with autistic children need social support for coping with stress and attunement due to having a child with developmental disabilities (Meral et al. 2012).

- **Siblings:** The siblings of individuals with autism have a variety of adjustment, coping difficulties, and impaired intimate relationships with their affected siblings. Different studies on parental characteristics relay a concern for the perceived stress in the health of the family environment. Sibling behaviors of persons with ASD include their self-competence and experience of living with brothers or sisters with autism. The studies on sibling characteristics revealed a variety of influences on personality traits, and they accentuate that the interaction of variables comprises the environment of families with persons of autism (Smith et al. 2010). Research also indicates that siblings of children with autism are at risk of bearing the psychological and emotional brunt of growing up alongside a child with behavioral difficulties. Many siblings have felt that their parents perceived their needs as being secondary, with more time and attention given to the child with autism. While they may have a deep love for their sibling, they may also harbor feelings of resentment at the amount of time their parents are spending with the child with autism and feel that they are being mistreated. Thus, anger, embarrassment, and guilt are expected, as they feel very protective of their sibling. Siblings of children with autism are significantly more likely to experience depression than the general population. Besides psychological problems, exhaustion may affect siblings responsible for domestic tasks and physical care. Problems may also arise when the increased parental expectations are not accompanied by increased parental time or attention (Gupta and Singhal, 2005). Under the circumstances, some of the parents avoid getting the second child if the first one is autistic.

Challenges for Parents and Families in Raising Autistic Children

- **Financial Stress:** Autism can place financial strains on families in several different ways. Some families spend fortunes on therapies and treatment for their children. The diagnosis of autism begins a journey that places profound demands on the family's human and financial resources for the remaining lifetime of the child. Autism is a biologically based developmental disorder that impairs an individual's ability to communicate, build relationships, and relate appropriately to the environment. Diagnosis is usually made in early childhood through a multidisciplinary assessment of behavior, developmental level, and communication ability.

  The efficacy of early intervention depends on the specific nature and severity of autism. Intervention strategies are expensive and require long hours of one-on-one interaction with a trained therapist or the use of costly foods or drug supplements. Health insurance falls far short of covering these needs. Special education services do not fill the gap either. Although public schools are legally obligated to provide a fair and appropriate education to children with autism, the educational programs that are provided are rarely sufficient to address the needs of school-aged children with autism and are not available to young adults with autism. Despite higher costs, most parents are forced to seek out and try early intervention strategies for their child's future. Costs associated with having a child with autism are not only limited to the cost of interventions. Like any other form of childhood disability, parents of a child with autism often face more significant outlays of time and money than they would for a neurologically typical child. Additional costs are also associated with extracurricular activities for children with disabilities. Health insurance may sometimes cover the cost of medical tests used in the diagnostic process and the cost of prescription medication. However, it will not pay for behavioral or other types of therapy for autism (Sharpe and Baker 2007).

- **Marital Maladjustment:** Marriages of some parents of children with developmental disabilities are portrayed as complex, dysfunctional, and particularly likely to end in either separation or divorce. Parents of children with disabilities experience more marital stress and discord than parents with normal children.

Families with autistic children face many stressors and challenges; today's partnership in marriage is more challenging and more complex than in the past years, especially for couples with special needs children (Al Horany et al. 2013). Marital stress around the child usually starts when one or both parents realize the child is not developing correctly. Couples with a child who does not seek their attention in the usual way, that is, eye contact, reaching out for or giving affection, seeking comfort when hurt, feel rejected or unimportant to the child. For those whose child develops commonly and then regresses around 18–24 months, there is the added loss of the child they knew slipping away. When a couple looks forward to having a child, and each person has an idea of what the expected child would be like, but the child does not match the expectation or regresses, the parent feels a loss and anguish.

- Under the circumstances, a marriage takes time to remain healthy, and all too often, time gets swallowed up by the autistic child's needs. Many children with ASD have difficulty sleeping, and at least one of the parents is sleep-deprived. In most cases, a role division occurs as one parent, usually the mother, becomes the autism expert while the father works harder to earn money or opts out. Consequently, the father becomes frustrated at the demands of the mother to interact or play with a child who does not know how, and mothers become frustrated at the lack of involvement of their partners (Silice-Kira 2008). Because of the demands associated with caring for an autistic child, parents do not have personal time, which results in a weakened affectionate bond between parents, depression, withdrawal of one parent from caregiving responsibilities, or even divorce (Greeff and Walt 2010). Mothers usually wonder what they did wrong, taking medications during pregnancy, exercising too much, and allowing the child to be vaccinated, thus adding feelings of guilt to an already stressful situation. Eventually, the couple feels isolated because they feel it is hard to take an autistic child to people's homes and are uncomfortable inviting people over. The stress of dealing with autism and all it entails, the constant and necessary advocacy at school, fighting for services and support, added financial burden, and trying to handle behaviors and meltdowns at home becomes a

Challenges for Parents and Families in Raising Autistic Children

wedge pushing the parents further and further apart (Silice-Kira 2008).

- **Caregiving:** Caregiving to a child with ASD is no easy task. It comes with its own ups and downs, challenges, and stress. Taking care of children with ASD may be a full-time job for some families or parents, as every child is unique. Each child has their own set of issues, severities, etc. Single parents and nuclear families especially face stress on account of taking care of their children. They may often not have the support and assistance of other family members, joint families, or relatives linked to kinship ties, compounding their stress levels and making it a significant challenge.

- **Self-Care:** One major challenge for an autistic child's parent is health challenges. The daily struggles they face in terms of the child's caregiving take a toll on their physical and mental health. They may experience feelings such as anger, guilt, shame, and helplessness over their child's disability. Without the support of a paid caregiver, extended or joint family, or even close families, parents struggle to care for their child, perform well at a job or multiple jobs, manage their home, and be multi-taskers. This leaves them with little or no time for themselves. This could mean limited or no socializing, rest, exercise, hobbies, interests, etc. The person's identity is subsumed, with the primary focus being the care of the child with their unique complexities, which becomes a challenge for the parents' self-care.

- **Communication:** Verbal communication is a challenge for some children with ASD. For parents of such children, communication is a problem that compounds the stress and anxiety of parents. Parents face the challenge of their children being unable to communicate their needs and wants. With children sometimes unaware of nonverbal communication and cues, parenting challenges get compounded. Under the circumstances, parents often experience communication problems with their autistic children. Many times, children who have autism do not know how to communicate with their parents and what they want or need, and other times, these children do not feel comfortable doing so.

Difficulty in communication can lead to frustration for both the parent and the child. As a result, parents of children with severe autism are unable to communicate with them at all.

- **Personal Health Care:** Mental health challenges of an autistic child's parent make them susceptible to other health challenges like depression, cancer, and an increased risk of early death. Thinking about the child's development and future may also lead to anxiety, fear, and psychological distress. The level of the disability and severity of the symptoms are major health stressors. A child with low cognitive development and functional abilities may exhibit behavior difficulties, which might be frustrating and overwhelming for their parents.

- **Behavioral Issues:** It can be frustrating and challenging to deal with a child who has severe behavioral problems, such as aggression and irritability. This is often one of the most challenging parts of parenting a child with autism. They may have outbursts and tantrums where they hit themselves or others, scream uncontrollably, and bite themselves or other people.

Behaviors are also inadvertently or accidentally reinforced by the caregiver. Caregivers sometimes ignore or give in to behaviors to avoid a tantrum, such as giving in to a request for food or not knowing how to help with fecal smearing. They may also reward negative behavior by letting the child stay up late or watch TV when behaving inappropriately.

- **Social Interaction:** A common issue that parents face when raising children with autism is related to social interaction. Many children who have autism do not know how to interact with other people, especially in social settings outside of the home. These interactions can be complex for the child and the parent, who often must help the child behave appropriately. Not knowing how to interact socially can make it difficult for children with autism to make friends or be accepted by their peers.

Challenges for Parents and Families in Raising Autistic Children

- **Organizing Household:** Due to the behavioral issues that children with autism often have, it can be difficult for parents to maintain a clean and organized home. Cleaning up after an autistic child who is having an outburst or tantrum is very challenging, as they may destroy parts of the house or throw things around in frustration. When this happens, organizing and cleaning the mess can be impossible.

    It is not just during a tantrum that organizing and cleaning are difficult. Many children with autism often have difficulty focusing on or taking part in daily chores such as making their bed, tidying up toys, picking clothes to wear, and caring for their hygiene. This can make it challenging to maintain a clean, organized home.

- **Maintaining Time:** Parents often do not have enough time for themselves, and this is especially true when they are raising a child with autism. This may be because parents spend much of the day caring for their children, planning activities and therapies, or just trying to keep them occupied. In addition to not having enough time for themselves, many parents neglect their own needs to care for their children. As a result, the parents become overwhelmed and exhausted, leaving little time or energy for themselves.

- **Sleepling at Nights:** It is estimated that as many as 60 percent of parents with children who have autism have trouble sleeping at one point or another. This lack of sleep can result from the child's frequent nighttime awakenings, bedwetting, talking in their sleep, or nightmares. It can also be due to hyperactivity during the day, making it difficult for children to calm down and fall asleep. It is important for parents not to neglect their own needs for sleep, as a lack of sleep can make them irritable and cause them to be less patient with their children. Parents should remember that they need healthy sleep to function correctly.

- **Stigmatization:** As there are many people on this planet, there are as many reactions as possible toward autism. Not everyone is sensitive, kind, or accepting of the autistic child like other normal children. Adverse reactions impact the child personally and the parents; the effects linger for some time, unfortunately, and thus challenge the parents of autistic children.

- **Get Support from Relatives:** Many parents of autistic children feel like they lack support from family members and friends when raising their children. Many times, relatives and friends do not understand the challenges that parents face in raising a child with autism, and this can lead to them not offering much help or support. It can also lead to them not understanding why things are done a certain way and treating the child as if they do not have autism.

  It is not only with family members and friends that parents lack support. Some parents need more support from their employers or teachers, causing them to miss work or school for long periods to care for their children. This can strain the family's finances and cause problems at work if they cannot make up for the missed time.

- **Social Isolation:** The parents of autistic children hesitate to communicate or participate in any social gathering like ceremonies, festivals, and so on. The parents feel that they are isolated from social activities, and some of the parents believe that their children are autistic because of the misdeeds of their forefathers in the past. Some of the parents reported that the neighbors and relatives do not want to interact with them due to the autism of their children because autism is a divine punishment for misdeeds.

Concluding Remarks

Autism spectrum disorder (ASD) is a complex neurological disorder that causes impairments in multiple areas of development, including social interaction, communication, and behavior. It typically appears within the first three years of life. Families with ASD children face extreme challenges in dealing with the behavioral problems associated with the disorder. The presence of an autistic child in a family has adverse effects on marital adjustments, sibling relationships, and daily family routines. Besides the parenting stress accompanying the disorder, it has substantial financial implications. Parents who have autistic children experience periods of disbelief, deep sadness, depression, self-blame, and guilt, whereas others

Challenges for Parents and Families in Raising Autistic Children

experience helplessness, feelings of inadequacy, anger, shock, and shame. Family members of children with autism are often perceived to experience adverse psychological effects, which may include a higher risk for depression, social isolation, and marital discord. The siblings of children with autism have a variety of adjustment, coping difficulties, and impaired intimate relationships with their affected siblings—the financial resources required for the medical and therapeutic intervention heavily burden families in several ways. The diagnosis of autism places profound demands on family human and financial resources for the remaining lifetime of the child. Because of the demands associated with caring for an autistic child, parents do not have personal time, which results in a weakened affectionate bond between parents, depression, and withdrawal of one parent from caregiving responsibilities or even divorce.

Raising a child with autism can be a challenging task for parents. There are many common issues that parents face when trying to raise a child with autism. Some of these issues include communication problems, behavioral issues, and struggles with social interaction. Parents often have to deal with a lot of stress and frustration when trying to care for a child with autism. However, there are ways that parents can help their children overcome these challenges and lead happy and successful lives.

References

Al Horany, A. K., S. A. Hassan, and M.Z. Bataineh. (2013). "A Review on Factors Affecting Marital Adjustment among Parents of Autistic Children and Gender Effects." *Life Science Journal*, 10(1): 120–132.

Charman, T., and G. Baird. (2002). "Practioner Review: Assessment and Diagnosis of Autism Spectrum Disorders in the Pre-school Years." *Journal of Child Psychology and Psychiatry*, 43(3): 289–305.

Cox, A., K. Klein, T. Charman, G. Baird, S. Baron-Cohen, J. Swettenham, S. Wheelwright, and A. Drew. (1999). "Autism Spectrum Disorders at Twenty and Forty-Two Months of Age: Suitability of Clinical and ADI-R Diagnosis." *Journal of Child Psychology and Psychiatry*, 40 (3): 719–732.

Dumas, J. E., L. C., Wolf, S. N., Fisma, and A. Culligan. (1991). "Parenting Stress, Child Behavior Problems, and Dysphora in Parents of Children with Autism, Down Syndrome, Behavior Distress, and Normal Development." *Exceptionality*, 2(2): 97–110.

Dunlap, G., K. Dyer, and R. L. Koegel. (1983). "Autistic Self-Dyches, T. T., L. K. Wilder, R. R. Sudweek, F. E. Obiokor, and B. Algozzine. (2004). *Multicultural Issues in Autism. Journal of Autism and Developmental Disorders*, 34(2).

Dyson, L. L. (1997). "Families of Young Children with Handicaps: Parental Stress and Family Functioning." *American Journal on Mental Retardation,* 95(6): 623–629.

Ecker, J. (2010). "Cultural Belief Systems in Autism and the Effects on Families." Cultural Psychology.

Gabriels, R. L., M. L. Cuccaro, D. E. Hill, B. J. Ivers, and E. Goldson. (2005). "Repetitive Behaviors in Autism: Relationship with associated Clinical Features." *Research in Developmental Disabilities,* 26(2): 169–181.

Gray, D. E. (1993). "Perceptions of Stigma: The Parents of Autistic Children." Sociology of Health and Illness, 15(1).

Greeff, P. A., and K. J. Walt. (2010). "Resilience in Families with an Autistic Child." *Education and Training in Autism and Developmental Disabilities*, 45(3): 347–355.

Gupta, A., and N. Singhal. (2005). "Psychosocial Support for Families of Children with Autism." *Asia Pacific Disability Rehabilitation Journal*, 16(2): 143–155.

Hoppe, S. E. (2005). "Parent Perceptions: Communication, Interaction, and Behavior in Autism." *Teaching Exceptional Children Plus*, 1(4): 43–55.

Ingersoll, B., and D. Hambrick. (2011). "The Relationship between the Broader Autism Phenotype, Child Severity, and Stress and Depression in Parents of Children with Spectrum Disorders." *Research in Autism Spectrum Disorders*, 5(1): 337–344.

Kesari, C., M. and Sigman. (1997). "Linking Parental Perceptions to Interactions in Young Children with Autism." *Journal of Autism and Developmental Disorders*, 27(1): 115–124.

Koegel, R. L., L. Schreibman, L.M. Loos, and H. Dirlich Wilhelm. (1992). "Consistent Stress Profiles in Mothers of Children with Autism." *Journal of Autism and Developmental Disorders*, 22(2):205–216.

Kourkoutas, E., V. Langher, R. Caldin, and E. Fountoulaki. (2012). "Experiences of Parents of Children with Autism: Parenting, Schooling, and Social Inclusion of Autistic Children." *Expanding Horizons*, Current Research on Interpersonal Acceptance.

Lecavalier, L., S. Leone, and J. Wiltz. (2006). "The Impact of Behavioral Problems on Caregiver Stress in Young People with ASD." *Journal of Intellectual Disability*, 50(3):172–183.

Leekam, S., J. Tandos, H. McConactie, E. Meins, K. Parkins, C. Wright, M. Turner, B. Arnold, L. Vittorini, and A. A. Couteur. (2007). "Repetitive

Behaviors in Typically Developing Two-Year-Olds." *Journal of Child Psychology and Psychiatry*, 48 (11):1131–1138.

Lord, C., and A. Pickles. (1996). "Language Level and Nonverbal Social-Communication Behaviors in Autistic and Language-Delayed Children." *Journal of the American Academy of Child and Adolescent Psychiatry*, 35 (3):1542–1550.

McCubbin, H. I., and J. M. Patterson. (1982). *Family Adaptation to Crises*. In H.I. McCubbin, A. E. Cauble and J. M. Patterson (Eds.). Family Stress, Coping, and Social Support. London: Charles C Thomas Publishers.

Meral, B. F., and A. Cavkaytar. (2012). "A Study on Social Support Perception of Parents Who Have Children with Autism." *International Journal on New Trends in Education and Their Implications*, Volume 3, Issue 3,

Prince, S. (2007). "Stress, Coping, and Psychological Well-Being: The Development of Resource Manual for Parents of Autistic Children."

Sharpe, D. L., and D. L. Baker. (2007). "Financial Issues Associated with Having a Child with Autism." *Journal of Family Economic Issues*, 28 (2):247–264.

Silice-Kira, C. (2008). "The Effects of Autism in Families and Partner Relationships." *American Association for Marriage and Family Therapy*, 12(3):45–52.

Stimulation and Intertrial Interval Duration". *American Journal of Mental Deficiency*, 12 (2): 88–202.

Whitaker, P. (2002). "Supporting Families of Preschool Children with Autism: What Parents Want and What Helps." *Autism*, 6(4): 411–426.

Chapter 10

PROBLEMS FACED BY AUTISTIC CHILDREN AT THE FAMILY LEVEL

Introduction

Most of the research on autism spectrum disorder (ASD) has been conducted in developed as well as affluent English-speaking countries around the West, which have extensive professional support services (Sharpe and Baker 2011). Initial research on autism diagnosis and service delivery in developing countries has suggested that diagnosis can be a cumbersome and frustrating process. Access to effective therapeutic services is often limited or nonexistent, and the more significant part of the burden of care rests on family members (Al-Salehi et al., 2009; Daley, 2002). Research is essential to finding effective ways to lessen the disease burden. The research on autism in developing countries, especially in Bangladesh, is meager.

Raising a child with autism involves an increase in the number of parental responsibilities or even leads to a change in parents' plans for their lives, which undoubtedly affects their attitude toward a child, relationships between spouses, and their physical and mental health. Identifying parental attitudes toward a child is vital because these attitudes shape the offspring's future development and personality. Therefore, this research aims to recognize parental attitudes toward their autistic children, indicate corrective actions if undesirable attitudes are identified, and put research results into practice. The main focus of this chapter is to explore the problems autistic children face at the family level in a kinship network system.

Autism and Related Problems

Children with difficulties or differences in relating and communicating may fall within a broad spectrum of diagnoses or challenges that includes language processing disorders, attention disorders, sensory or regulatory disorders, and autism spectrum disorder. These challenges often involve several different underlying difficulties, including the following:

- **Taking in Sensations or Information:** The child may be under or overreactive to the information received through their senses of vision, hearing, touch, smell, taste, and body awareness.

- **Processing Information:** The child may have difficulty understanding or organizing the sensory information they receive.

- **Planning or Executing Responses:** The child may have trouble using their body or thoughts to respond to the information they have received.

A child may develop unusual or concerning behaviors in response to these difficulties or differences. For example, a child may be so under-reactive to the sensation that they spin in circles in an attempt to increase their sensory input; another child, overwhelmed by the confusing information they have received about their world, may withdraw, finding security in lining up their transports over and over again. Examples of behaviors parents may observe by area of difficulty are the following:

Felt Unpleasant Emotion

Individuals with autism spectrum disorders experience difficulties associated with an inadequate appreciation of social-emotional cues, as shown by a lack of responses to other people's emotions, poor use of social signals, and weak integration of social, emotional, and communicative behaviors. For example, autistic children might feel all negative or unpleasant emotions, such as anger, not recognize when they are excited, or label all feelings that are hard to describe as being bored.

Language Communication

A child or adult with autism spectrum disorders may have problems with social interaction and communication skills, including any of these signs: failure to respond to their name or appearance, not being able to hear at times, resistance to cuddling and holding, seeming preference for playing alone and retreating into their world.

Regulatory and Sensory-Motor

Regulation is the ability to change arousal to match the environment and the activity. Essentially, it is the ability to adjust to an optimal level of arousal. Throughout the day, the brain and body constantly do things to increase and decrease arousal levels and regulate them. Sometimes, it is called self-soothing. Some children with autism have more difficulty regulating themselves than others. This could include trouble with sensory regulation or emotional regulation. Difficulty with regulation is often reported in autism.

Self-Stimulatory Behaviors

It includes spinning, hand flapping, and head banging. A child receives a diagnosis based on observation of the behaviors outlined above. However, though a child may share a common diagnosis with other children, each has a unique pattern of development and functioning. Each child is unique in sensory and other information processing and motor planning, that is, the ability to plan and carry out actions. Some children overreact to sensations like touch and sound, while others are under-reactive. Some children have relatively strong auditory memories and can memorize entire scripts; others have relatively solid visual memories. Some children can plan several actions, such as going upstairs, getting a toy, and returning it. In contrast, others can only carry out one action at a time, becoming very fragmented in their behavior.

In addition to differences in sensory processing and motor planning, children differ in their essential mastery of the foundations for relating, communicating, and thinking. Some children with ASD can form relationships and engage in two-way communication, while others appear to be very self-absorbed and aimless. Some children can focus and attend and engage with others but can only participate in a back-and-forth flow of communication in a limited way, finding it difficult to use language meaningfully or connect ideas for logical and reflective thinking. Other children show some mastery of the basics and the ability to engage in more complex communication, create ideas, and use them logically. However, they are very limited in applying these abilities to various situations. Therefore, while some children may exhibit common symptoms that lead to a diagnosis of an autistic spectrum disorder, their patterns and, thus, their paths toward recovery are pretty varied.

Problems at the Family Level

Caring for a family member with autism costs money and places a burden on family finances. On the other hand, children with autism in the developed world are generally enrolled in regular or special educational institutes for their skills development training so that they can stand on their own. It should be noted that the number of special education institutes for autistic children is meager in Bangladesh, and most of the institutes are situated in urban areas where only 30 percent of people live. Moreover, special education for autistic children in Bangladesh is expensive, and as a result, a significant percentage of them are under the protection of family. It has been reported that only the parents take a keen interest in caring for their autistic offspring compared to the other members, including siblings. It is found that autistic children are being abused in different ways, viz. physically, emotionally, and sexually at the family and community levels, either by the parents or the persons who relate to the kinship network system and the community people.

- **Physical Abuse:** Physical abuse is the intentional infliction of injury by beating, punching, kicking, biting, or otherwise upon children. Hosking and Powel (1985) mentioned that the history of child abuse is long, but there was little interest in this subject until the 1960s. Physical abuse has commonly been defined as an act of commission by the parents along with the other members of the family and is characterized by nonaccidental injury and infliction of overt physical violence (Kelly 1983; Wolf 1988). Physical abuse usually occurs in discrete, low-frequency episodes and is often accompanied by frustration and anger toward the child (Kelly 1983). Physical abuse may take place in multi-natural ways. Rogger et al. (2005) noted that specific physical abuse is common among autistic children, but it may happen in different forms and different natures. It is caused by a person's inability to control anger (Sarker and Khan 2009). Physical abuse is injury ranging from minor bruises to severe fractures or even death. It includes punching, beating, kicking, biting, shaking, throwing, stabbing, choking, hitting with a hand, stick, strap, or other objects, burning or otherwise harming a child. Such injury is considered abuse regardless of whether the parents or caretakers intended to hurt the child.

- **Emotional Abuse:** Emotional abuse is a pattern of behavior that impairs a child's emotional development or sense of self-worth. This may include constant criticism, threats, rejection, and withholding of love, affection, support, or guidance. Emotional abuse is often difficult to prove; therefore, it may not be able to intervene without evidence of harm to the child. Teyber (1992) argued that sadness and anger generate an emotional reaction in children that leads to depression. On the other hand, emotional abuse of children is associated with family violence. Family violence includes spouse abuse, child abuse, sibling abuse, and parent abuse. The nature of severe violence is kicking, biting, punching, hitting or trying to hit with an object, beating, and threatening with a knife that fueled the mindset for emotional abuse of the children (Gelles and Straus 1988). Emotional abuse occurs when the parents or guardians cause severe emotional injury by repeatedly terrorizing or berating a child.

- **Sexual Abuse:** Sexual abuse of children refers to sexual behavior between a child and an adult or between two children when one of them is older or more dominant. The sexual behaviors include touching breasts, buttocks, and genitals, whether the victim is dressed or undressed; exhibitionism; fellatio; and penetration of the vagina with sexual organs. Sexual abuse is defined as the persuasion, inducement, enticement, or coercion of any child to engage in or assist any other person to engage in any sexually explicit conduct or simulation of such conduct to produce a visual depiction of such conduct or the rape and, in cases of the caretaker or inter-familial relationships, statutory rape, molestation, prostitution, or other form of sexual exploitation of children or incest with children. Emotional abuse is almost always present when other forms are identified. Victims experience both short- and long-term psychological effects of rape. Studies over the decades have consistently demonstrated that rape victims often experience significant sy anxiety, depression, and post-traumatic stress (Green and Pomeroy, 2007). Rape has other specific psychological effects. Sexual abuse is also associated with rape, and the effects of rape can arise from forced sexual assault. Its frequency causes visible bruising or bleeding in and around the vagina. The rape can have many other physical consequences.

- **Child Neglect:** Child neglect is the failure to provide adequate care and protection for children. Physical neglect may involve failure to provide basic needs in terms of food, clothing, medical care, and education, along with the inability to protect the child from danger. The most extreme form of neglect leads to the syndrome of failure to thrive.

- **Stress for Autistic Child**: The stress of caring for an autistic child is both natural and acute. Parents are more stressful for their children than other types of handicaps. However, fathers of children with disabilities, in comparison to mothers, have higher levels of stress associated with the child's communication abilities and their feelings of attachment to the child. In this study, 44.44 percent of mothers of children with autism reported some symptoms of physical and psychological tension. Fathers seem to have some of the same troubles as mothers, but they cannot express it. Most of the fathers in the study expressed concern about the well-being of their wives due to the excessive burden.

Problems Faced by Autistic Children at the Family Level

Anxiety of the Autistic Children

Anxiety is a normal part of development, but research confirms that people with autism experience elevated levels of anxiety in comparison to their typically developing peers. An extensive review of the literature by White et al. (2009) revealed that up to 84 percent of individuals with autism meet the criteria for clinically diagnosed anxiety disorders.

Due to characteristic communication difficulties, an autistic person may have severe anxiety issues but have a decreased ability to express it. As noted by Howlin (1997), the inability of people with autism to communicate feelings of disturbance, anxiety, or distress can also mean that it is often challenging to diagnose depressive or anxiety states. Anxiety may manifest in an autistic person through the following:

- Social phobia
- Excessive worry or rumination
- Obsessive-compulsive behavior
- Hyper-vigilance or seeming shell-shocked
- Phobias in general
- Avoidance behaviors
- Rigid routines and resistance to change
- Stimming and self-injurious behavior
- Controlling behaviors – oppositional defiance
- Meltdowns
- Shut down

Challenges to Autistic Children

It is revealed in this study that autistic children face challenges in everyday life. The depth of challenge depends upon the level of autism. It should be mentioned that some challenges are more complex than others. People who are diagnosed with autism can have difficulty making and keeping relationships because it is harder for them to understand the feelings of others, and it is hard for them to know what others need. Not only is it hard for people with autism to develop relationships, but speech and verbal communication can be difficult for them as well, which can also make it hard for them to carry on a conversation. Some autistic individuals can excel in one particular subject, whereas other autistic individuals take the intelligence test and score below the average.

- **Inability to have a Social Circle:** Autistic children are restless around people. They are rattled when people interact with them. This is because their communication skills do not develop like other children. They are unable to understand thoughts and feelings and can not express themselves. This makes them fidget when people try to interact with them. They may seem to ignore, hide away, or sometimes reach out angrily. If the child is found alone in a group or shying away from people, make sure he keeps track of his social activities.

- **Irritability and Uncontrolled Anger:** A child as small as 18 months old might not have legitimate life issues to feel frustrated. Therefore, if the child is constantly irritated, it could be because of some underlying irritation. The inability to express and understand the basic rules might rue the child. Finding themselves being different from people around them can stress them. This could lead to severe mood swings, and it may get serious as they grow up.

- **Difficulty in Following Instructions:** Children with autism have difficulty following instructions. They show annoyance toward basic day routines. Because of broken communication, the flow of activities in their heads breaks, making them unable to follow a pattern. For instance, the first thing to do after getting up in the morning is go to the washroom, wash your hands, and then brush. They might now understand the relevance of doing three activities in a proper flow. They do not take it as a tantrum or disobedience if it prevails for long.

- **Hatred for a Particular Object:** As autistic children do not consider themselves one of the groups, they may develop ideas of their own. They could relate these ideas and thoughts to a specific object or a person. Depending on the concept they have created, they may have a special attachment or extreme hate for the object. For instance, they can relate to a toy, which may make them feel comfortable and loved.

- **Delay in Language Acquisition:** Language development is often delayed in children with autism, and the language that does develop is deficient in conversational use and predominantly nonverbal. Under these circumstances, the child with autism fails to grasp the meaning of communication and has difficulty comprehending gestures and speech. The child makes little social use of communication skills and has a deficit in social imitation. Coupled with this difficulty is the child's misinterpretation of facial expressions.

  A child with autism usually has delayed speech or normal development until two years, when it ceases. The speech that the child with autism does develop tends to have an oddity in vocal volume and pitch. It has been reported that fifteen out of twenty parents of their children with ASD show delays in nonverbal communication and spoken language. They may have words that they use to label things but never request things. They may have unusual words for their overall language level, such as saying letters or numbers when they do not yet have names they use for family members. Most young children go through a phase where they repeat what they hear. Children with ASDs may repeat for a more extended period and repeat conversations with the tone of voice in which they heard them.

Daily Life Challenges

The daily life challenges are almost common that are faced by autistic kids. Unfortunately, most children are not diagnosed with autism until three years of age. Some of the common problems faced by autistic children were found in the research area under study. These problems are explained here.

- **Repetitive and Stereotyped Play:** Repetitive actions are one of the main diagnostic criteria of autism. However, they are not uniquely associated with autism. Some of the parents reported that repetitive actions have long been recognized as a standard component of mental disturbance. Stereotypes are involuntary movements that are rhythmic, repetitive, and purposeless. These may include rocking, head nodding, or self-injurious behaviors, which are also stereotyped and repetitive but differ in that they can potentially cause harm to the child. These may include hitting, biting, and scratching. Compulsions are purposeful behaviors that are repetitive and performed according to rules. These include ordering, checking, hoarding, and so forth.

- **Conversational Problem:** Children with autism cannot carry on a conversational interchange of thoughts and information about the same topic with another person. Teachers have reported that 90 percent of autistic children cannot continue conversations with others. Autistic children cannot maintain sequence during interaction with others.

- **Problem of Contact:** A few autistic children initiate play with other children, and they are usually unresponsive to any who may approach them. Autistic infants may avert their gaze if parents try to communicate with them, and they are described as engaging in less eye contact than their peers. The sheer amount of gazing may sometimes be relatively average, but not how it is used. Normal children gaze to gain someone's attention or to direct the other person's attention to an object, but autistic children generally do not.

- **Problem of Rigid Behaviors:** People with autism display rigid behaviors, including stereotypical, self-injury, compulsion, ritual, sameness, and restriction. Studies have revealed that about 50 percent of parents face rigid behaviors in their children at home and outside. About 60 percent of teachers have said that they face rigid behaviors in autistic children when they teach them.

- **Loss of Social Skills:** Loss of social skills is another problem faced by children with autism. Parents have observed that sometimes an autistic child may seem to lose social skills that they once had, such as waving goodbye. This study found it in about one out of four cases.

Problems Faced by Autistic Children at the Family Level

- **Imitative Action:** For instance, when someone chants in front of them, they start to recite. Parents and teachers reported that autistic children try to imitate other gestures and language activities.

- **Problem of Hearing:** In the research areas, about 15 to 20 percent of autistic children suffer from hearing problems. About 20 percent of parents reported that their children have hearing problems. On the other hand, teachers said that ten autistic children face hearing problems, but they are not deaf.

- **Sleeping Problem:** Children with ASD tend to have problems falling asleep or staying asleep or have other sleep problems. Babies ease into a regular sleep cycle and wakefulness during the first few months of life. They gradually reduce the number of daytime naps they need and start sleeping for more extended periods at night. Parents have reported that their children continue to have difficulty falling asleep or sleeping through the night, and the problem can persist long after children start school.

- **Dietary Problem:** Not all children are habituated to the same food habits. Many of them are incompetent in chewing. Some of them suffer from dental complications, which impede eating. Some vomit when the meat piece is more significant than the average size they are used to. Unusual eating behavior occurs in about 30 percent of children with ASD, to the extent that it was formerly a diagnostic indicator. The most common problem is selectivity, although eating rituals and food refusal also occur.

- **Lack of Understanding:** It is difficult to understand children's demands or designs when they express themselves outside their language. This research has found that about eight out of twenty parents face an understanding problem with their children.

- **Epilepsy:** Many have epilepsy, which is an internal physiological disorder that, in its motion, makes them feel sleepy or asleep. It is interesting to note that about five parents reported that their child has epilepsy.

- **Educational Problem**: Education is one of the problems in schools for autistic children. The majority of children with autism never reach a high level of attainment. Around half of all children with autism have severe to moderate learning problems. Because of this, many education authorities argue against placement in highly specialized autistic provisions when places are readily available in schools for children with more general learning disabilities.

- **Problem of Peer Relationships:** The child with autism has a reduced capacity for shared attention and fails to develop skills to attract other people's attention. This is presented in the failure to establish normal peer relationships, the avoidance of visual or physical contact, and the behavior of the child with autism toward people as if they were objects. Children with autism often are unsuccessful at building developmentally appropriate relationships with their peers. This results in part from a perceived indifference to the interests of others, which is frequently demonstrated.

Concluding Remarks

The mothers reported the explored problems the autistic children faced at the household level because the autistic children could not communicate with others, and they were not even willing to communicate either verbally or symbolically. The identified problems are isolation from others, aggression, stress, and depression. Sometimes, they are a victim of domestic violence in the kinship network system, especially by the siblings, which includes physical torture like slapping, biting, kicking, kneeing another room alone with a lock and key when visitors visit the family, and non-cooperation in daily life, and so on.

It has been reported by the mothers that their autistic children are deprived of love and affection by the family members and relatives who are very important to them. Some mothers said their children are not invited or even allowed to participate in social festivals or gatherings. Most of the time, the relatives and neighbors want to keep away from them. This negligence is painful for the parents and the children as well. This negative attitude of the neighbors and relatives put the children in isolation.

References

Al-Salehi, S. M. (2009). "Consanguineous Marriage in Saudi Arabia: Presentation, Clinical Correlates and Co-morbidity. *Transcult Psychiatry*, 46(2):340–347.

Bittles, A. (2008). "Consanguinity and Its Relevance to Clinical Genetics." *Clinical Genetics.* 9(2): 89–98.

———. (2001). "Consanguinity and Its Relevance to Clinical Genetics." *Clinical Genetics*, 60(2): 89–98.

Bittles, A. H. and Black, M. L. (2010). "Evolution in Health and Medicine Sackler Colloquium: Consanguinity, Human Evolution, and Complex Diseases." *Proceedings of National Academic Science*, 107 (1):1779–1786.

Fareed, M., and M. Afzal. (2016). "Increased Cardiovascular Risks Associated with Familial Inbreeding: A Population-Based Study of Adolescent Cohort." *Annals of Epidemiology.* 26 (4): 283–92.

Grant, J. C., and A. H. Bittles,. (1997). "The Comparative Role of Consanguinity in Infant and Childhood Mortality in Pakistan." *Annals of Human Genetics*, 61(1):143–9.

Green, D., S. Chandler, T. Charman, E. Simonoff, and G. Baird. (2016). "Brief Report: DSM-5 Sensory Behaviors in Children with and without an Autism Spectrum Disorder." *Journal of Autism and Developmental Disorders*, 46(11):3597–606.

Heidari, F., S. Dastgiri, and N. Tajaddini. (2014). "Prevalence and Risk Factors of Consanguineous Marriage." *European Journal of General Medicine*, 1(4):248–255.

Hoskin, G., and R. Powel. (1985). *Chronic Childhood Disorder.* Bristol: John Wright and Sons Ltd.

Howlin, P. (1997). "Outcome in Adult Life for Individuals with Autism," in F. Volkmar (ed.) Autism and Developmental Disorders. New York: Cambridge University Press.

Kelly, J. A. (1983). *Treating Child Abusive Families: Intervention based on Skills Training Principles*. New York: Plenum Press.

Prayson, A. S. (2016). "Autism, Genetics and Inbreeding: An Evolutionary View." *Journal of Public Health and Epidemiology*, 8(5): 67–71.

Rogger, P., V. Mangiaterra, F. Bustreo, and F. Rosati. (2005). "The Health Impact of Child Labor in Developing Countries. Evidence from Cross-Countries Data." *American Journal of Public Health*, 97 (2): 271–275.

Sandridge, A. L., J. Takeddin, E. Al-Kaabi, and Y. Frances. (2010). "Consanguinity in Qatar: Knowledge, Attitude, and Practice in a Population Born between 1946 and 1991." *Journal of Biosocial Science*, 42(2):59–82.

Sarker, Profulla C. (2015). "Consanguinity, Inbreeding and Their Impact on Reproductive Health and Human Development in Inbred Communities." *The Indian Journal of Anthropology*, 3 (2): 69–80.

Wolf, D. A. (1988). "Child Abuse and Neglect." In E.J. Mash and L.G. Terdal (eds.), *Behavioral Assessment of Childhood Disorders*. New York: Guilford Press.

Chapter 11

INITIATIVES OF GOs, NGOs, AND POs ABOUT AUTISM SPECTRUM DISORDERS

Introduction

The Government of Bangladesh has already made a strong political commitment to reducing the stigma related to autism spectrum disorders (ASD) and its management. The Ministry of Primary and Mass Education has developed a short episode of the *Meena* cartoon to raise awareness of autism and staged an interactive famous theater in 158 upazila (sub-district) on the issue of autism. In June 2010, the Center for Neurodevelopment and Autism in Children (CNAC) was inaugurated, and ten Shishu Bikash Kendra (Child et al.) were developed in the medical colleges and other specialized centers. Moreover, the government initiated seventy-three Disability Service Centres at district and upazila (subdistrict) levels, with a special Autism Corner. Autism is already incorporated into the primary education curriculum. In addition, an autism-related chapter has been included in the book *Physical Teaching, Health Science and Sports* for grades nine and ten. Moreover, knowledge of autism is provided in almost every grade. It was an essential step in combating the stigma against autism among parents, relatives, neighbors, and the general masses (Assaf and Khawaja 2009).

Autism spectrum disorder (ASD) is a complex and highly heritable neurodevelopmental disease that is characterized by individuals with a combination of behavioral and cognitive impairments (Clark et al., 2009). ASD is directly linked with consanguineous marriages, which are widely practiced in inbred communities, keeping in view the quasi-socioeconomic interests of both the groom and bride families. However, they do not think about the fate of the future generation that they might be the victims of autism. The GOs, NGOs, and INGOs did not take any initiative to prevent autism by discouraging cross-cousin and parallel-cousin marriages. Consanguineous marriage is not the absolute cause of autism in the offspring, but there is a possibility of autism in the offspring due to inbreeding. Even the Government of Bangladesh did not take any initiative to discourage consanguineous marriages, which may be one of the causes of autism in the inbred community of Bangladesh. Consanguineous marriages are already strictly prohibited in many developed and developing countries across the world to prevent autism spectrum disorder (ASD) and, at the same time, to make their citizens assets instead of liabilities (Sarker 2015; Rogers and Lewis 1989).

Action Plan against Autism

The government has developed a strategic action plan for children with special needs under inclusive education. All children with autism can get twenty minutes extra time in public examinations. There are two percent reserved seats for admission for autistic children in the private sector. Moreover, the National Autism Academy was established under the Ministry of Education to conduct substantial research to develop culturally sensitive, cost-effective, and intervention-based curricula and contents (Center for Research and Information 2014). In addition, Bangladesh hosted the most significant regional conference on autism in July 2012. At the meeting, the Dhaka Declaration on autism spectrum disorders was ratified by seven regional countries. They were addressing the socioeconomic needs of individuals, families, and societies affected by autism spectrum disorders, developmental disorders, and associated disabilities at the United Nations General Assembly in 2013, which was unanimously adopted. A One Stop Mobile Service program is running to reach families living in villages concerned about accessibility to medical services. The government uses electronic, print, and social media, donates huge funds, develops new infrastructure, and involves celebrities and national and international political figures for proper attention to autistic children. Social media sites like Facebook play an important role in other electronic media. Facebook pages, support groups, and video clips helped to connect and share the successful stories of autistic children. Every year, on the second of April, the Ministry of Health and Family Welfare (MoHFW) observes World Autism Awareness Day. All these measures help in reducing the stigma related to autism.

Programs for Autism

Since the independence of Bangladesh in 1971, the Constitution has mandated equality, non-discrimination, and the creation of equitable measures for all those who are underprivileged. Therefore, all programs and services for autism and other disabilities are under its jurisdiction. Besides, the government is fully aware of the prevalence of autism, and it is one of the first countries to become a party to the UN Convention on the Rights of Persons with Disabilities and Its Optional Protocol.

The government has implemented many revolutionary programs to build an autism-friendly Bangladesh, which is regarded as a milestone for this segment. Parents of autistic children, civil society members, non-state actors, NGOs, media, and the general people need to come forward to make the government initiatives sustainable and prosperous. Consequently, the parliament of Bangladesh has promulgated two necessary acts to protect the rights and ensure the safety of the differently able persons. One act is the Disability Rights Law, 2013; the other is the Neurodevelopmental Disability Protection Trust Act, 2013. However, in many cases, the acts are hardly implemented in the case of autism because of stigma, lack of concern initiative, and less political commitment at the local level. On the other hand, the Neurodevelopmental Disability Protection Trust Act of 2013 highlights the issues related to providing physical, psychological, and economic assistance to all persons with disabilities like autism, their nurture, security, and rehabilitation to ensure their social empowerment and focus on the development of pertinent education system and knowledge paradigm. Both within the country as well as in the global context, Bangladesh is playing a commendable role in undertaking appropriate policies, social awareness, and intervention programs to mitigate the emerging and increasing problem of autism.

The Disability Rights Law ensures the rights and dignity of persons with disabilities by stipulating twenty-one rights. Rights to educational, physical, and psychological improvement, rights to participation in social and state activities, rights to get the national identity cards and be listed in the voters' roll, mandates enrolment in regular schools, reservation of seats on all forms of public transportation, accessibility provisions in all public places, including retrofitting, equal opportunities in employment, and protection of inherited property rights are few of the rights.

Services to the Autistic Children

Customizing the programs and planning based on Bangladesh's culture, social expectations, financial and professional resources, and infrastructure is equally important. Autism is a relatively recent discovery in Bangladesh. The trained parents are now operating the special schools. The medical-based diagnosis system in Bangladesh has started to identify autistic children through the child development center of government child hospitals. Bangladesh needs more and more specialist physicians, special educators, psychologists, and therapists to confront the issue comprehensively. Conjointly, adequate screening for autism, culturally and linguistically appropriate interventions, scientifically based academic programs in inclusive settings, appropriate job training, and sheltered accommodations for young adults with disabilities are the significant future challenges for Bangladesh, like any other country of the world.

Acts Mitigating Autism

The honorable prime minister of Bangladesh, Sheikh Hasina, said that the Awami League government had passed the Neurodevelopmental Disability Protection Trust Act of 2013, Neurodevelopmental Disability (NDD) Protection Trust Act of 2015, Protection of Rights of Persons with Disabilities Act of 2013 for the Welfare of All Persons with Disabilities, including persons with autism. In addition, the Bangladesh Rehabilitation Council Enacted Act of 2018 and Disability Special Education Policy of 2019. The honorable prime minister said that appropriate action plans have been adopted to implement all these laws successfully. Apart from this, Neurodevelopmental Disorders Chairperson Saima Wazed's initiative, advice, and relentless efforts have created a broad awareness at the national, regional, and international levels to improve the quality of life and well-being of children and individuals with autism.

The prime minister said that the government of Bangladesh has already formulated the National Strategy and Action Plan 2016–2030 to protect the rights of people with disabilities. Under this action plan, people with autism and disabilities are being provided with all necessary services at different stages of their life Cycle. The NDD *Suraksha* (protection) Trust has already provided online training to parents and guardians on home-based care and mental health care for children and individuals with autism. This protection trust also works on hotline-based medical services, digital telemedicine services, and curriculum formulation for school students.

Pointing out that the program of establishing fourteen autism and NDD service centers as a pilot project in fourteen places in the country under the NDD Protection Trust is underway in the current financial year (2022–23), Prime Minister Sheikh Hasina said that through these centers, children and individuals with autism and other NDDs will be provided with social and medical procedures at various stages of their life cycle. It should be noted that the multidisciplinary team will give about seventeen types of services, including early intervention of international standards. This program will be gradually expanded throughout the country. Besides, the establishment of eight medical, education, and rehabilitation centers in eight divisions for children and persons with NDD characteristics is underway (American Psychiatric Association 2013).

Bangladesh in Global Setting

Bangladesh is commendable and active in undertaking appropriate policies, social awareness, and intervention programs to mitigate the emerging and increasing autism problem. The honorable prime minister of Bangladesh, Sheikh Hasina, has taken a keen interest in bringing this issue forward nationally and globally. Some of the proactive roles of the Government of Bangladesh include the formation of the South Asian Autism Network (SAAN) and the preparation of its Charter.

In July 2012, Bangladesh hosted the most significant regional conference on autism, during which seven regional countries ratified the Dhaka

Declaration on autism spectrum disorders. Bangladesh tabled Resolution 67/82, addressing the socioeconomic needs of individuals, families, and societies affected by autism spectrum disorders, developmental disorders, and associated disabilities, at the United Nations General Assembly in 2013, which was unanimously adopted. Bangladesh was also the one to initiate the WHO resolution titled "Comprehensive and Coordinated Efforts for the Management of autism spectrum disorders," proposed by the state of Qatar at the WHO Executive Board meeting held in May 2013, which was adopted unanimously. Saima Wazed Hossain, a school psychologist and global advocate for autism, has been actively engaged in international and domestic advocacy of mental health disabilities. She has been a significant champion for the cause of autism and assisted in mobilizing executive board members at the WHO Secretariat to support this resolution (Actions Speak Louder than Words: Bangladesh Unique Approach to Addressing the Public Health Challenge of ASD 2014).

The World Health Organization recently honored Saima Wazed for her outstanding contributions to autism spectrum disorders. She is among the first two recipients of the newly instituted Award for Excellence in Public Health, conferred by the WHO regional director for the Southeast Asia Region, Dr. Poonam Khetrapal Singh. Dr. Singh commended Saima Hossain as the driving force behind Bangladesh's leadership in advancing the cause of autism in the region and worldwide. Her work has helped to build multidisciplinary and multi-stakeholder partnerships for ASDs and childhood development disorders, which resulted in the adoption of resolutions at the United Nations and the World Health Organization (Hamamy and Bittles 2009).

According to the World Health Organisation, Bangladesh is a global leader in raising awareness regarding autism. The government has undertaken various programs concerning autism, which is commendable. This volume has already mentioned that the Government of Bangladesh has also promulgated two necessary acts that concern individuals with autism and help protect their rights and ensure their safety—the Disability Rights Law of 2013 and the Neurodevelopmental Disability Protection Trust Act of 2013. However, as experts have opined, the country cannot yet provide optimal treatment and support to those who have autism, especially in terms of having enough treatment centers that specialize in treating autism.

As the prime minister rightly said in her address marking the eleventh World Autism Awareness Day, those who have autism should in no way be neglected by society, as they, too, are a part of it and may have much more talent than the average person. Moreover, by adequately harnessing those talents, we, as a society, can indeed benefit greatly. We hope the government will continue its excellent work raising awareness about autism. Moreover, we urge it to work more proactively with the private sector to set up additional treatment centers for people with autism.

Observance of National Autism Day

Bangladesh is regarded as a role model in autism awareness and rehabilitating people who have autism. Bangladesh has taken pioneering steps to overcome service barriers for individuals with autism. No other country in the Southeast Asian region has committed itself quite so strategically to developing systems that address the needs of persons with autism and the problematic situation faced by their families. The country is also being recognized globally as an exemplar for combating autism with measures to register childbirths and raising awareness at the national level on the role of the family in the psychological and physical nourishment of autistic children. The government's political will and pioneering initiatives are praiseworthy, but the legacy needs to be translated into sustainable strategies, multidisciplinary planning, and evidence-based actions.

National Advisory Committee

Ms. Saima Wazed, chairperson of the National Advisory Committee on Autism, said that the committee involves international experts apart from a few Bangladeshi experts. It is a small body, but four task forces will work on advocacy and awareness, education, service delivery, and research. Under the circumstances, Prime Minister Sheikh Hasina said, "If the potential of children and adolescents with autism is identified and raised in a humane environment with proper care, education, training, and love, they will also become assets of the family, society, and the state. We are determined to turn Bangladesh into a developed, prosperous, smart Bangladesh by 2041, along with everyone in the society."

National Policy on Autism

Bangladesh has formulated a national policy for persons with disability. Bangladesh has ratified some important social protection-related agreements in the United Nations Convention. Accordingly, the concerned Ministry has formulated a National Plan of Action to implement the provisions of the said convention. Some important conventions are the United Nations Convention on the Rights of the Child 1991, the Convention on the Elimination of All Forms of Discrimination against Women (CEDAW), 1984, Convention on the Rights of Persons with Disabilities 2007. The government has decided to Ratify the Optional Protocol on the Rights of Persons with Disabilities; on 4 May 2008, the United Nations General Assembly designated April 2, 2008, as the first World Autism Awareness Day. Coincidentally, the National Disability Day of Bangladesh fell on the same day. For the first time, the autism issue was placed in an oversized shape and raised awareness about autism among the mass people.

It is to be noted that Bangladesh has initiated many things to deal with autism. The country is regarded as a role model in raising autism awareness and rehabilitation of people who have autism. It has taken pioneering steps to overcome service barriers for individuals with autism. No other country in the South Asian region has committed itself quite so strategically to developing systems that address the needs of persons with autism and the problematic situation faced by their families. The country is also being recognized globally as an exemplar for combating autism with measures to register childbirths and raising awareness at the national level on the role of the family in the psychological and physical nourishment of autistic children. Nevertheless, this is a critical period in the history of disability and neurodevelopmental disability in Bangladesh. The government's political will and pioneering initiatives are praiseworthy, but the legacy needs to be translated into sustainable strategies, multidisciplinary planning, and evidence-based actions.

Both within the country as well as in the global context, Bangladesh is playing a commendable role in undertaking appropriate policies, social awareness, and intervention programs to mitigate the emerging and increasing problem of autism. Since the independence of Bangladesh in 1971, the Constitution has mandated equality, non-discrimination, and the creation of equitable measures for all those who are underprivileged. Therefore, all programs and services for autism and other disabilities are under its jurisdiction. Besides, the government is fully aware of the prevalence of autism, and it is one of the first countries to become a party to the UN Convention on the Rights of Persons with Disabilities and Its Optional Protocol. Bangladesh has formulated many policies, especially the national policy for persons with disability, 1995 for social protection and ensuring the rights of vulnerable groups. Bangladesh has ratified some important social protection-related agreements in the United Nations Convention.

Autism School and Therapy Center

An adequate number of autism schools and therapy centers with all facilities for treatment and therapies are essential for the development of autistic children. About a percent of children have autism around the world. It is assumed that the figure would be more than that in Bangladesh. However, an adequate number of good-quality autism schools and therapy centers are not available in Bangladesh to accommodate the significant number of autistic children. Most of the autism schools do not have enough facilities for effective treatment and therapies. Moreover, the existing autism schools in the country are costly compared to the regular schools. Consequently, a significant percentage of children with autism are deprived of treatment, therapies, and special education. Recently, only a few autism schools and therapy centers have been established in urban areas by the government, NGOs, and some autism-affected families. The names of the autism schools and autism centers established in different parts of the country are given below.

There are eighty-three schools and therapy centers in Bangladesh for autistic children. Among these institutes, a few are Advanced School for Special Children, Advanced Learning and Special School, *Alokito Shishu* Treatment Based School, *Alokito Shishu* Treatment Based School, *Amar Joti* Special School, Angels Care Foundation, Angel Foundation for Children with Special Needs, Angels of Heaven, Autism Bangladesh, Institute of Neurodevelopment and Research, Autism Care and Advancement Center, Autism and ADHD Care Center, Autism in Bangladesh, Autistic Children'sWelfare, Blue Bird Special School, Beautiful Mind, Bongo

Bondhu Community Clinic-Autism Center, and so on. All the school deals with autistic and other neuro-related children between the ages of 2.5 to 10. The teaching includes Applied Behavior Analysis (ABA), Picture Exchange Communication System (PECS), Individualized Education Plan (IEP), and other scientific approaches recommended by the specialist therapist. Different therapies, like speech, occupational, sensory integration, and physiotherapy, are available in one-to-one methods. These therapies are applied by well-trained, expert, and experienced therapists (Khlat, 1997).

Concluding Remarks

Private organizations (POs), nongovernmental organizations (NGOs), and voluntary organizations (VOs) work either individually or in partnership with INGOs for autistic children in providing special education and therapy. The establishment of adequate autism schools and therapy centers by the government is essential to accommodate many autistic children in the country. Society's rich people can also come forward for noble jobs. The autism school should have enough facilities for the treatment and therapies of the children. The therapies are to be made free of cost or very cheap. Rural and urban areas are to be considered while establishing autism schools and therapy centers to make autistic children self-dependent. These schools and therapy centers may be non-governmental, nonprofitable, nonpolitical, voluntary, or charitable organizations. These are therapy-based special needs schools established keeping in view to providing education and treatment and generating awareness about autism in society, aiming to increase acceptance and promote a friendly environment and rehabilitation for autistic children to integrate with the mainstream of the population.

References

American Psychiatric Association. (2013). Diagnostic and Statistical Manual of Mental Disorders. Arlington: American Psychiatric Publishing Ltd.

Assaf, S. and M. Khawaja. (2009). "Consanguinity Trends and Correlates in the Palestinian Territories." *Journal of Biosocial Sciences*, 41(1): 107–124.

Center for Research and Information. (2014). Global Autism Movement and Bangladesh, Dhaka: CRI.

Clark, C. J., A. Hill, K. Jabber, and J. G. Silverman. (2009). "Violence during Pregnancy in Jordan: Its Prevalence and Associated Risk and Protective Factors." *Violence against Women*, 15(6): 720–735.

Hamamy, H., and A. H. Bittles. (2009). "Genetic Clinics in Arab Communities: Meeting Individual, Family, and Community Needs." *Public Health Genomics*, 12(1): 30–40.

Khlat, M. (1997). Genetic Disorders among Arab Populations. New York: Oxford University Press.

Rabbani, M., A. Helal, M. Mannan, W. A. Chowdhury, and M. F. Alam. (2014). "Autism in Bangladesh: Window for Stigma Removal." Dhaka: Report of the International Meeting for Autism Research.

Rogers, S. J., and H. Lewis. (1989). "An Effective Day Treatment Model for Young Children with Pervasive Developmental Disorders." *Journal of the American Academy of Child and Adolescent Psychiatry*, 28(2): 207–214.

Sarker, Profulla C. (2015). "Consanguinity, Inbreeding, and their Impact on Reproductive Health and Human Development in Inbred Communities." *The Indian Journal of Anthropology*, 3(2):69–80.

Wang, P., C. Michaels, and M. Day. (2011). "Stresses and Coping Strategies of Chinese Families with Autism and Other Developmental Disabilities." *Journal of Autism Development Disorders*, 41(3): 783–795.

Chapter 12

Life Cycle-Focused ASD Prevention and Rehabilitation Strategy

Introduction

Autism spectrum disorder (ASD) is a neurodevelopmental condition characterized by deficits in social communication, social interactions, and restricted, repetitive patterns of behaviors, interests, or activities (American Psychiatric Association, 2013). ASD is a highly heterogeneous condition with the concept of a spectrum capturing the differences among autistic people in terms of symptoms, intelligence and language abilities, neuropsychological underpinnings, cognitive style, information processing, sensory deviations, etiology, and comorbidities, as well as the levels of functioning, adaptation, and well-being. Before the prevention strategies, the way autism is formed evolves over the lifetime of each, and it needs to be conceptualized, which will contribute to determining the ways and timing of preventive interventions. Studies revealed that autism spectrum disorder (ASD) could also result from effects derived from environmental risk factors.

A deeper understanding of epigenetics has underscored the conceptualization of disorders as a mismatch between an individual and a specific environment rather than an abnormality per se. It can explain autism as an expected reaction to a non-optimal environment for the individual in a physical and psychosocial context (Hens 2019). Specifically, in ASD, it is hypothesized that genetic and environmental factors lead to a subject's atypical patterns of interactions with the environment, with impaired engagement in social interactions. These risk processes will result, on the one hand, in abnormal social and linguistic brain circuitry and, eventually, mediate the development of full-blown ASD (i.e., autism will create itself). On the other hand, they may intervene through epigenetics in the expression of the susceptibility genes, further strengthening their effects, as if in a vicious cycle (Dawson 2008). Finally, as one would expect, the overall outcome of the disease and its burden is further determined by social, psychological, and biological factors from childhood to adolescence and adulthood through constant feedback loops between the environment and the disorder indices.

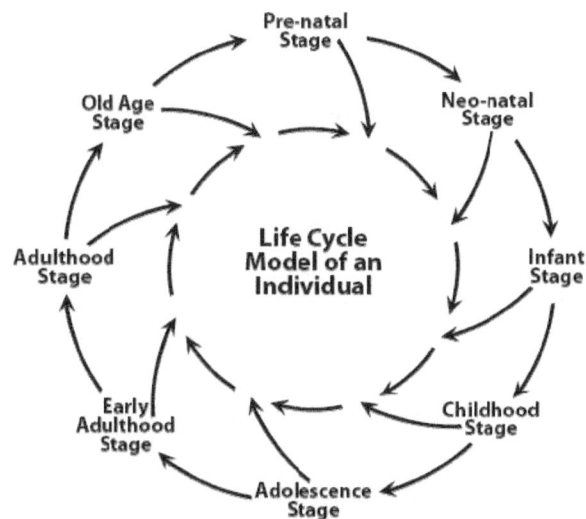

Fig. 7: Spiral Model of Life Cycle of an Individual

Stages of the Human Life Cycle

Human life is divided into eight stages: prenatal, neonatal, infancy, childhood, adolescence, early adulthood, adulthood, and old age. All of these stages of life have physical, emotional, social, and cultural network relationships, which start from the embryonic stage and continue to old age (Sarker 2022). The first five stages of life cycles are under the care and protection of parents or guardians along with other members of the family who are interlocked in kinship ties, either in consanguineal or affinal relationships. It should be noted that the consanguineal relationship is an inborn relationship that takes place by birth, and the affinal relationship is by marriage (Sarker 2017). In the sixth and seventh stages of the life cycle, the individuals become independent or self-dependent, stand on their own, and usually take responsibility for dependents based on their socioeconomic and cultural systems. In the last stage, the individuals become dependent on the children, the state, or any other foster or charitable organization.

Life Cycle-Focused Prevention Strategy

Although human life is divided here into eight specific stages, these stages are converted into preschool to the prepubertal stage, childhood to adulthood stage, older children and adolescents, transition to adulthood, and adulthood to old age. All these stages have individual identities; the prevention strategies have developed but are interlinked. Commonly, the prevention of autism spectrum disorder (ASD) can be distinguished into three forms.

- The first one is a primary prevention that aims to reduce the incidence of a disorder and target the broad population.
- (The next one is a secondary prevention that targets the selected at-risk groups aiming to reduce the prevalence of the disorder or its severity.
- Thirdly, it is tertiary prevention for indicated subjects to preserve functional adaptations and the person's well-being and avoid relapses (Rudenstine and Galea 2015).

These strategies should be applied in a life course approach, from the prenatal period to old age, with a variable focus for each type depending on the age of the targeted subjects due to the conceptual overlap between the types of prevention and the population they target (e.g., a primary intervention could target an at-risk population only), as well as that of secondary and tertiary preventions with actual treatment interventions, a more productive framework could be to dissect prevention in mental health based on the time the relevant measures are taken.

In this framework, and based on the development of autism described above, primary prevention for autism would mean efforts, preconceptionally and during pregnancy, to manipulate its root causes in an attempt to increase resilience and reduce occurrence (Hertz-Picciotto et al. 2018; D'Arcy and Meng 2014). These targets are the developmental risk and preventive factors known to participate in the etiopathology of ASD in the interplay with genetic causes. During the first two-to-three years of life, prevention measures, secondary or tertiary, will be aimed at altering the developmental cascade that started before birth (Bonnet-Brilhault et al., 2018) and, thus, alleviating or even preventing the emergence of autistic symptomatology (Dawson, 2008). From childhood and adolescence until adulthood and old age, and with ASD fully present, prevention strategies are mainly at the secondary and tertiary levels in an attempt to increase or preserve the level of adaptation and the well-being of the autistic person. Furthermore, they will prevent the appearance of secondary problems, such as highly disruptive behaviors, depression, and transition difficulties. In a broad sense, all treatment interventions for these ages display an inherited preventive value. This chapter discusses the possibilities for prevention efforts during these three periods of the life of an autistic person based on the available data.

Strategy before Conception

Genetic and environmental factors have already been identified as the main reasons for autism in different studies across the East and the West. This chapter explores how these strategies must be executed before the conception of offspring. The root causation of ASD is multifactorial, with multiple genes interacting with each other and with environmental factors (American Psychiatric Association, 2013). Genes represent the baseline susceptibility, but epigenetic phenomena derive from a 'toxic environmental load' and act during the right critical time window (Loomis et al. 2017). Consequently, physiological changes that overcome the individual's resilience and adaptation finally translate into a neuro-atypical phenotype (Werling and Geschwind 2013). In this context, prevention seeks the optimal manipulation of these factors that can render the causal constellation insufficient to produce the ASD phenotype or at least the full-blown one (Doshi-Velez et al. 2014).

The second category of factors represents prevention targets for the general population, as their effects extend beyond the ASD pathobiology, and prevention measures should be addressed for the whole population. According to the "prevention paradox," the expected benefits on the incidence of ASD of such effective large-scale prevention measures can outperform the ones from measures aiming only at the high-risk subpopulation (King et al. 2014; Rogers et al. 2019). The following prevention strategies are interlocked with each other in sociocultural, bio-psychological, genetic, and environmental issues of the individual with autism spectrum disorder (ASD). The couple should implement these strategies before being a child.

- **To Avoid Consanguineous Marriage:** Consanguineous marriage should be avoided before the bridegroom and bride selection, whether previously connected with kinship ties or parallel-cousin or cross-cousin relationships. Suppose they are identified as related to either a first cousin, second cousin, or even third cousin. In that case, they need to be involved in marriage to avoid the inbreeding of their offspring. This may be one of the leading causes of autism due to gene mutation with the same blood group as well as the same genetic pole.

- **To Avoid Spousal Age Gap:** The parental age indicates that older fathers, older or very young mothers, and increased age differences between parents increase the risk of ASD (Navarro-Pardo et al. 2021). Many studies revealed that the spousal age gap between 8 to 10 years is allowed, which does not genetically affect the autism of their offspring. In South Asian society, traditional marriages allow a more extended age gap between the husbands and the wives, especially if the husbands are older than the wives, irrespective of religion and ethnicity.

- **Assisted Reproductive Technology (ART):** Similarly, Assisted Reproductive Technology (ART) is often a mandatory choice to address a couple's infertility. Albeit concerns from clinicians, the role of ART in the risk of ASD is not yet prominent, especially when ART is examined as a whole (King et al. 2014).

- **Intracytoplasmic Sperm Injection:** Specific relevant treatments, for example, intracytoplasmic sperm injection, may have a greater additive risk for ASD (Dworzynski et al. 2012). The assessment of the possible risk for ART becomes more pertinent if the techniques are used for gender selection, given the substantially higher incidence of ASD in boys and the higher recurrence risk for boys in the presence of a sibling already diagnosed with ASD (Johnson and Myers 2007).

- **Gender Preference of Offspring:** The overall reduction in risk by gender selection choosing a female is calculated as 3 percent if the couple has one autistic child and 15 percent if they have two autistic children (Reichow et al. 2012). The residual risk for ASD from gender selection could be increased to the extent that ART itself increases the risk of ASD, while an increase in congenital disabilities and other adverse pregnancy outcomes related to ART should also be one of the factors in the decision.

- **Ethical Issues Need to Be Considered:** Ethical issues are also pertinent to this "preventive" approach (Reichow et al. 2012). Overall, gender selection seems more rational when the risk reduction is substantial, as in the case where there are already two autistic siblings, and it is less attractive when the risk reduction is less (e.g. when there is just a positive family history of ASD).

- **Congenital Hypothyroidism:** Congenital hypothyroidism is implicated in mental disabilities and may be in the pathophysiology of ASD (Zwaigenbaum and Penner 2018), but it was recently shown that maternal hypothyroidism during pregnancy also increases the risk of ASD (Dover and Le 2007). Testing for congenital hypothyroidism is a well-established practice in most countries that should be coupled with relevant testing during pregnancy.

- **Air and Chemical Pollutions:** Air and chemical pollution are also a public health matter. Data for the effect on ASD risk due to air pollution, that is, hazardous air pollutants and air pollutants criteria as defined in the Western countries, and endocrine-disrupting chemicals like those found in pesticides, plastics, and fragrances are inconclusive (King et al. 2014; Doshi-Velez et al. 2014). However, studies with more sophisticated designs for actual exposure measurements have implicated some pesticides (Doshi-Velez et al. 2014). Interestingly, prenatal pesticide exposure can be mitigated by a higher folic acid intake in the first month of pregnancy (Maestro et al. 2002).

- **Maternal Smoking:** Maternal smoking during pregnancy is correlated with risks for pregnancy and birth complications, which include miscarriages, decreased growth, complications during labor, preterm birth, stillbirth, and sudden unexpected death in infancy (Yirmiya and Charman 2010) as well as long-term effects like asthma and behavioral problems. Several meta-analyses reported noncontribution to autism spectrum disorder (ASD) risk, but in more sophisticated analyses of confounding factors like second-hand smoking and the severity of smoking, a positive correlation is revealed (Penner et al. 2018; Blank et al. 2020). Smoking cessation programs have to be implemented during pregnancy, particularly in women from a lower socioeconomic status.

- **Premature Birth:** Apart from the multiple consequences of reduced or increased fetal growth and preterm deliveries on the general health of the child, a higher prevalence of ASD has been systematically reported in children born prematurely as well as in those with bilateral deviances in fetal growth (Shaw et al. 2020). It is not clear if these are risk factors per se or the expression of other factors, but general measures for the optimal clinical care of pregnant women should be applied to reduce their incidence (Ozonoff et al. 2018). Relevant to these, studies consistently report a higher prevalence of pregnancy complications and obstetric suboptimality in children with ASD, including pre-eclampsia (Green et al. 2016; Yates and Le 2016). However, it seems more possible that this could be rather an epiphenomenon of ASD or the result of a shared risk factor.

- **Maternal Obesity and Gestational Diabetes:** Maternal obesity and gestational diabetes, along with other metabolic conditions that elevate glucose, triglycerides, cholesterol, leptin, and proinflammatory immune markers, may substantially increase the risk for ASD (Robins et al. 2009; Pandey et al. 2008). Relevant follow-up and treatment programs should also be applied to reduce ASD risk and prevent short—and long-term health risks for the mother, developing fetus, and offspring (Robins 2008).

- **Immune Reactions:** A literature review has found that immune deficiency in the mother during the embryonic stage of the fetus may be a risk factor for autism in the offspring. Immune reactions during pregnancy represent additive risk factors, whether the results of infections, with congenital rubella being the historical paradigm or maternal autoimmune conditions (Baduel et al. 2017; Campbell et al. 2017).

- **Maternal Influenza:** Maternal influenza and other viral infections in the first trimester, as well as bacterial infections and prolonged fever in the second trimester, increased the risk of ASD up to threefold. These latter data could explain the seasonality of the births reported in several studies and vitamin D levels or pesticide use (Myers and Johnson 2007). Toward mitigating the risk of ASD, general preventive measures to avoid infections should be implemented on a whole population level. For mothers at high risk for ASD, vaccination programs should be offered, especially for such well-established risk infectious factors as rubella. At the same time, a more aggressive treatment of the fever should be clinical practice (Lord et al. 2020).

- **Shortage in Inter-Pregnancy Interval:** Shortage of interpregnancy intervals of about 60–84 months has also been associated with a higher ASD incidence (King et al. 2014; Doshi-Velez et al. 2014). Thus, a shortage of interpregnancy intervals should be avoided in high-risk families. In one case, intense supplementation with vitamins, folic acid, and minerals and generous nutrition intake during the new pregnancy could play a protective role against autism in offspring.

- **Nutrient Deficiencies:** Nutrient deficiencies like vitamin D, iron, and polyunsaturated fatty acid, especially omega 3, have also less robustly been correlated with a higher risk for ASD (King et al. 2014). Iron is a critical mineral for brain development and functioning, but the data from two studies on the specific risk for ASD are contradictory (Doshi-Velez et al. 2014). Omega-3 supplementation or fish consumption is associated with a higher IQ and better neurodevelopment, but its correlation with ASD is unclear (ibid). However, an extensive prospective study showed that higher fish fat consumption prenatally had a protective effect on ASD, even after controlling for the mercury levels bioaccumulating in them (Kossyvaki and Papoudi 2016).

- **Constraints of Maternal Folic:** Maternal folic acid supplementation is a standard preventive measure proposed by many international authorities like the CDC in the USA to prevent neural tube defects; its connection to ASD is less conclusive in the literature (Whitehouse et al. 2017). However, some studies reported significant protective effects around conception, especially in inherent inefficient folate metabolism (Zwaigenbaum et al. 2009).

- **Problem of Breastfeeding:** Studies revealed that ASD may be associated with those babies who do not get adequate breastfeeding in their infant stage. The probability of ASD may be reduced through adequate breastfeeding of the offspring for up to one year. Research data has shown that children with ASD were significantly less likely to have been breastfed (Shivers and Plavnick 2015).

Rehabilitation Strategies

Rehabilitation is a relative term, and this term was used by the International Labor Conference in 1995 to mean restoring disabled persons to the fullest possible physical, mental, social, vocational, and economic usefulness of which they are capable (Taylor and Taylor 1970). Inamdar and Parajpe (1981) state that rehabilitation is restoring forfeited rights and privileges. In the concept of Waldman (1982), rehabilitation is the combined and coordinated use of medical, social, educational, and vocational measures for training the individual to the highest possible level of functional ability.

Life Cycle-Focused ASD Prevention and Rehabilitation Strategy

In the context of autism spectrum disorder, rehabilitation means restoring the working ability in different phases of the life cycle to utilize the total capacity to become productive members of society through income-generating programs. More specifically, rehabilitation means restoring the neuro-psychosocial and economic condition of autistic people by providing skill development training for employment to make them active members of society (Sarker, 2017). Rehabilitation strategies are confined here to neuro-psychosocial measures and skill development training, starting from preschool to the pubertal stage, childhood to adulthood stage, older children and adolescents, and adulthood and old age.

- **Preschool to Prepubertal Stage:** This section deals with the strategies between the preschool and the pubertal stage of the life cycle of the autistic child. A detailed individual plan should be the basis of all the chosen components of the intervention, depending on the strengths and weaknesses of the person and with clear short and long-term goals. In principle, these extremely diverse intervention efforts have the following common preventive goals:

    ➢ **Communication and Social Skills:** Protect future autonomy at the highest possible level through increasing communication, social skills, and daily living skills. Continuation of the interventions from the previous stage, intensive behavioral interventions and especially those with developmental components like the Naturalistic Developmental Behavioural Intervention (NDBI) or the Social Communications or Emotional Regulation or Transactional Support (SCERTS), the Treatment and Education of Autistic and related Communication Handicapped Children (TEACHC) program and a plethora of other targeted interventions such as social skills, speech and language and occupational therapies claim to target increased adaptation (Bremer et al. 2016; Sanchack and Thomas 2016).

    ➢ **Avoid Emergence of Challenging Behaviors:** Avoiding the emergence of challenging behaviors is one of the strategies to prevent autism in the early stage of life of autistic children. This could be the result of interventions assuring that communication abilities meet the respective needs—for example, the use of a Picture Exchange Communication System (PECS); dealing with the sensory needs and deviances, for instance, Sensory Integration Therapy and Diet (SITD), relevant environmental accommodations, etc.; and increasing the predictability to reduce anxiety (e.g., with the use of visual schedules, calendars, and other visual cues). It is fundamental toward this preventive goal to identify at an early stage and deal with common medical and psychiatric comorbidities and conditions, such as general health and pain, seizures, constipation and other gastrointestinal (GI) symptoms, sleep problems, intellectual disability, learning disorders, bullying, anxiety (Paavonen et al. 2003; Phillips and Appleton 2004).

- **Parental Acceptance and Engagement:** Facilitate and preserve parental acceptance and engagement in the support of their children. Parental engagement is indispensable for parent mediating programs and professional-based ones to generalize the acquired skills and reduce financial and time encumbrances. However, parental training and psychoeducation should be delivered in various ways. Reduced adaptive adjustment acceptance and increased feelings of blame and despair critically influence the psychological, including anxiety, depression, and somatic well-being of the parent (Giannotti et al. 2006), impairing the parent's ability to participate effectively in the child's management and training. Thus, professional training *demands* to parents should always be accompanied by measures aiming at increasing acceptance and ensuring the well-being of the parents (Sanchack and Thomas 2016).

- **Academic Learning:** Attain academic learning commensurate with the individual's cognitive abilities. Although ASD is famously impersonated by people with savant skills and individuals with exceptional academic achievements, the reality is that there is considerable heterogeneity in their academic achievements, with a substantial danger of underperforming (Owens et al. 2005). The covering of the previously mentioned goals to obtain appropriate abilities and behaviors should be coupled with proper support—e.g., visual aids, extra academic or psychological sessions, prevention of bullying, and social skills training at school (Pasquali et al., 2011), etc.—and relevant educational and environmental accommodations to secure a successful inclusion in the appropriate for each child school setting (Sanchack and Thomas 2016).

- **Childhood to Adulthood Stage:** It has already focused on prevention strategies aiming mainly at reducing the incidence, prevalence, and severity of autism symptoms in this chapter, but we need to discuss the preventive measures to maximize and sustain adaptation (Bremer 2016). Adaptive functioning, although not wholly independent from autism (symptom) severity or IQ, is not determined exclusively by them but instead captures the transaction between an individual and their environmental contexts (Owen 2009). This is reflected in the severity classes in the DSM-5 that are based on the level of needed support (Kim et al. 2009). It is this support throughout the lifespan that can alter the rather adverse outcomes of autistic people in adulthood (Horvath and Perman 2002). Thus, any treatment, measure, or support offered from preschool to old age has a preventive component for the individual's overall quality of life.

- **Older Children and Adolescents:** Most previous goals continue to be pursued in this developmental period, but the interventions should be directed more toward specific solutions for the rising problems. There must be a continuation of care for the consistency of measures that should be taken. As the individual grows, there is an enormous diversity in the overall clinical picture, with some having more problems but others doing as well or even better (Kern 2001). Toward the end of primary school, there may be a tendency to reduce or stop specific interventions, especially as the family gets tired or the child is sometimes less willing to attend. However, this may have significant repercussions since light stresses. Thus, parents and professionals should be more cautious and meticulous in preparing individuals for changes to prevent behavioral relapses. Training and emotional support of the parents, either in groups or individually, should continue in this phase. The needs of their growing children are changing; for example, the emergence of sexuality and their own emotional needs continue to impact them and their relationships. Furthermore, the diagnosis and its implications should be reasserted frequently, as parents often tend to 'forget' this based also on their assumption of maturation by age or that they can grow out of it. According to a recent study, less than 0.5 percent of children lose the diagnosis of autism, with 6.5 percent more just losing it to another neurodevelopmental disorder (Plioplys 1998).

However, especially in higher-functioning individuals, more complex needs also emerge that can endanger the goals mentioned for the previous period, which include autonomy, avoidance of challenging behaviors, and academic achievements. These needs comprise the renegotiation of all established relationships, for example, a common need for adolescents, body changes, sexuality, and more complex peer relationships. There is no doubt about the prevention value of preparing the preadolescent individual with autism and their family for the upcoming body changes, the self-care and hygiene needed, and the new rules that must be followed to stay safe (DelGiudice-Asch 1999). The same holds for sexuality education, preventive measures for sexual abuse, and recognizing early signs of it, as well as exploring sexual orientation and identity (Granpeesheh 2010). There have been reports of a higher relevant diversity among people with ASD compared to their neurotypical counterparts (Elder et al., 2006).

During this period, and for a substantial part of high-functioning ASD individuals, although longing for social life and relationships is present, social and relationship-based difficulties tend to increase, leading to a more profound sense of isolation and frustration (Kuriyama et al. 2002). Social skills training can prevent further isolation of the individual and protect their future quality of life. Pertinent to the above are the related issues of self-esteem and the knowledge and acceptance of their diagnosis, both of which should be clear preventive targets through psychotherapy and psychoeducation (Adams and Holloway 2004). People with

ASD have lower self-esteem, endangering them further to other psychopathological manifestations, for example, depression, anxiety, etc. (Politi et al. 2004). On the other hand, knowing and coming to terms with their diagnosis is not only good practice but is often an imperative need for teenagers with high-functioning autism. The use of an appropriate strategy to do so can enhance ASD self-awareness without impairing self-esteem and prevent chronic frustration over a series of misconceptions and wrong assumptions about their difficulties (Politi et al. 2008).

A final preventive target for older children and adolescents is the meticulous screening for any comorbid psychopathology emerging during these rapidly changing years. In addition to the diagnoses reported to concur in the previous stage, an autistic can have disruptive, impulse control and conduct disorders, obsessive-compulsive disorder, bipolar disorders, and schizophrenia spectrum disorders. At the same time, depression and anxiety are more prevalent than before (Paavonen et al. 2003). Given the difficulty of recognizing these often-overshadowed additional symptoms, especially in lower-functioning individuals, a diagnosis can be missed with detrimental effects on the person's overall functioning. If, however, the comorbidities are noticed, suitable interventions should be implemented, apart from psychopharmacology cognitive-behavioral therapy (CBT) and mindfulness-based interventions (Delorme et al. 2013).

- **Adulthood and Old Age:** The main prevention target in this last period is achieving a good quality of life (QoL). Despite a successful transition to adulthood, pressing needs remain, as recently stated in relevant laws associated with the Autism Care Act or Autism Act. Based on these laws, the community is urged to take supportive measures for adults with ASD without intellectual impairment to expand and retain their autonomy and participation and to prevent mental and physical health deterioration (Bozdagi et al., 2013). Prevention for adult ages consists of the following measures.

> **Continuation of the Practical Measures:** The practical measures described for the transition period, including housing, employment, and social and everyday functioning, will continue through relative initiatives by the local community and support by the welfare system. Meaningful employment can improve the quality of life, offer structure, social inclusion and participation, financial stability and independence, upgrade housing and leisure activities, improve subjective well-being, and protect psychological and physical health (Sanchack and Thomas, 2016).

> **Enhancement of Social Skills:** Enhancing the social skills attained in the previous stages and their adaptation to the new age context. Social skills group interventions are effective at increasing social skills knowledge and social participation.

> **Comorbidities Vigilance:** This is also fundamental in this stage, as the prevalence of both physical and mental health conditions in adult life is high, regardless of the presence of intellectual disability. Persons with ASD present risk factors inherent to their diagnosis that, along with relevant environmental stressors, lead to more psychiatric symptoms, especially depression and anxiety.

These can be mitigated with preventive measures, such as programs that increase social participation and leisure activities before using medications. It is noteworthy that individuals with high-functioning ASD, especially women, report suicidal ideations and plans at higher rates than the average population or psychotics, and this is even in the absence of depression. Moreover, suicide is one of the leading causes of higher mortality rates in the ASD population, along with the elevated prevalence of general health problems from almost all systems, with neurological epilepsy being the most common. The increased prevalence of physical diseases leads to higher mortality and impacts the degradation of their QoL. The extent to which these higher morbidities and mortalities reflect an insufficient awareness and diagnosis from health providers and decreased help sought from the autistic population, as well as health and lifestyle ASD-related issues, show that they can be straightforward targets for prevention.

- **Transition to Adulthood:** The required additional interventions for this critical period aim to prevent the CDC-described dismal situation for young autistic adults: high rates of unemployment or underemployment and low participation in education beyond high school. At the same time, the majority continue to live with family members. This is particularly pertinent to those with higher cognitive ability. For the lower-functioning individuals, a clear plan should be drawn comprising educational and vocational parameters and living circumstances, their mental abilities and adaptive skills, their likes and dislikes, the parents' realistic expectations, and the available resources in the community. This plan can presuppose prevocational and vocational training, followed by a range of options from competitive employment with some support to work in sheltered workshops or day services and from semi-independent living with the backing of a supervised living environment. In the case of work in the community, they may need help in securing and training on the actual job, as well as liaising with employers and other employees and personal ongoing support to prevent adverse events that can lead to a loss of the job (Kolevzon et al. 2014).

It should be noted that things are more complicated for the individuals at the higher end of the spectrum, and measures should be introduced along the triptych of education, employment, and independent living. The first step should be a career counseling assessment by professionals with sound knowledge of both counseling and the disorder, using standardized assessment tools specifically designed for ASD, like the Autism Work Skills Questionnaire (AWSQ), and qualitative methods to overcome social communication difficulties to facilitate person-to-person job matching (Vahdatpour et al. 2016).

The next step, depending on the career decision reached by the individual and, to some extent, in collaboration with his family, could lead to further education on the relevant level, viz.

postsecondary vocational training, college, university, or directly to work placement. For the first part, the successful completion of further schooling, both academically and socially, needs supportive measures directed at the students, such as social planning and organization skills, and to the academic environment. The level and quality of such support offered in a few colleges and universities could underpin the difference between a successful and socially active autistic student and a dropout or someone frustrated and depressed (Sanchack and Thomas 2016).

The final challenge correlating with the previous ones for a successful transitional plan is independent living. Apart from the physical housing problem, independent living for people with ASD comprises a series of other important, relevant issues like tasks of day-to-day living, socializing, access to health and welfare services, and dealing with the criminal justice system (Bozdagi et al., 2013). There is a need for a systematic and thorough assessment of the overall adaptive skills of the person who is about to move out from his parental home, as well as of the available community resources to determine the type of independent living they will adapt to, that is type and location of residential arrangements, commuting needs, funding schemes, type and amount of support needed, and the therapeutic supporting team ... The final plan must be put together with the participation of the autistic person.

The above triptych represents the primary challenges in the transition to adult life. Successful settlement, along with the previously mentioned continuous needs, social skills, comorbidities, vigilance and treatment, and environmental accommodations, is the only way to a smooth transition to a successful and happy life.

Concluding Remarks

This chapter summarised the preventive opportunities for ASD within an individual's lifespan. There is evidence that primary prevention from the preconception period until the perinatal one can decrease the incidence of autism. However, given the intense variability in the quality of data published and the often-contradictory results presented, it is proposed the formation of a panel of experts with an ongoing assessment of the published data on the risk factors for ASD and the production of relevant state-of-the-art preventive guidelines for each one of them. Apart from the noticeable gains of such an endeavor, it will also facilitate the carrying out of more accurate prevention intervention trials.

Some researchers argue that all interventions throughout the lifespan have an inherent tertiary prevention quality against the goals by which their effectiveness should be measured. It should be noted that the critical component in this conceptualization is the increase of adaptive functioning, such as better behavioral and psychosocial functioning through a relevant compensation in skills, behaviors, and impairments, as well as through an increase in understanding and acceptance from their environment, viz. parents, school, peers and community. To be productive for and protective of the QoL of the person with autism, these interventions should be continuous, comprehensive, and coordinated, based on the developmental realities and needs of each phase, supported by the welfare system, and coupled with constant vigilance for medical or psychiatric comorbidities. Thus, prevention strategies should be a priority for researchers, advocates, stakeholders, and public health.

References

Adams, J. B., and C. Holloway. (2004). "Pilot Study of a Moderate Dose Multivitamin/Mineral Supplement for Children with Autistic Spectrum Disorder." *Journal of Alternative and Complementary Medicine*, 10(6):1033–9.

American Psychiatric Association, (2013). Diagnostic and Statistical Manual of Mental Disorders. Arlington: American Psychiatric Publishing Ltd.

Baduel, S., Q. Guillon, M. H. Afzali, N. Foudon, J. Kruck, and B. Rogé. (2017). "The French Version of the Modified-Checklist for Autism in Toddlers (M-CHAT): 'A Validation Study on a French Sample of 24-Month-old Children.'" *Journal of Autism and Developmental Disorders*, 47(2):297–304.

Ballaban-Gil, K., and R. Tuchman. (2000). "Epilepsy and Epileptiform EEG: Association with Autism and Language Disorders." *Mental Retardation and Developmental Disabilities Research Reviews*, 6(4):300–8.

Baranek, G. T. (1999). "Autism during Infancy: A Retrospective Video Analysis of Sensory-Motor and Social Behaviors at 9–12 Months of Age." *Journal of Autism and Developmental Disorders*, 29(3):213–24.

Bell, J. G., E. E. MacKinlay, J. R. Dick, D. J. MacDonald, R. M. Boyle, and A. C. Glen. (2004). "Essential Fatty Acids and Phospholipase A2 in Autistic Spectrum Disorders." *Prostaglandins, Leukotrienes, and Essential Fatty Acids*, 71(4):201–4.

Blank, M. S., J. B. Turner, P. W. Fisher, E. B. Guthrie, and A. H. Whitaker. (2020). "The Need for a Clinically Useful Schema of Social Communication." *Journal of American Academy Child Adolescence Psychiatry*, 59(11):1198–200.

Bonnet-Brilhault, F., T. A. Rajerison, C. Paillet, M. Guimard-Brunault, A. Saby, L. Ponson, G. Tripi, J. Malvy, and S. Roux. (2018). "Autism is a

Prenatal Disorder: Evidence from Late Gestation Brain Overgrowth." *Autism Research*, 11(4): 1635–1642.

Bozdagi, O., T. Tavassoli, and J. D. Buxbaum. (2013). 'Insulin-like Growth Factor-1 Rescues Synaptic and Motor Deficits in a Mouse Model of Autism and Developmental Delay'. *Molecular Autism*, 4(1):1–4.

Bremer, E., M. Crozier, and M. Lloyd. (2016). "A Systematic Review of the Behavioral Outcomes Following Exercise Interventions for Children and Youth with Autism Spectrum Disorder." *Autism*, 20(8):899–915.

Campbell, K., K. L. Carpenter, S. Espinosa, J. Hashemi, Q. Qiu, M. Tepper, R. Calderbank, G. Sapiro, H. L. Egger, J. P. Baker, and G. Dawson. (2017). "Use of a Digital Modified Checklist for Autism in Toddlers-Revised with Follow-Up to Improve Quality of Screening for Autism." *Journal of Pediatric*, 183 (3):133–9.

D'Arcy, C., and X. Meng. (2014). "Prevention of Common Mental Disorders: Conceptual Framework and Effective Interventions." *Current Opinion in Psychiatry*, 27 (3): 294–301.

Dawson, G. (2008). "Early Behavioral Intervention, Brain Plasticity, and the Prevention of Autism Spectrum Disorder." *Development of Psychopathology*, 20 (2): 775–803.

DelGiudice-Asch, G., L. Simon, J. Schmeidler, C. Cunningham-Rundles, and E. Hollander. (1999). "Brief Report: A Pilot Open Clinical Trial of Intravenous Immunoglobulin in Childhood Autism." *Journal of Autism and Developmental Disorders*, 29(2):157–60.

Delorme, R., E. Ey, R. Toro, M. Leboyer, C. Gillberg, and T. Bourgeron. (2013)." Progress toward Treatments for Synaptic Defects in Autism." *Nature Medicine*, 19(6):685–94.

Doshi-Velez, F., Y. Ge, and I. Kohane. (2014). "Comorbidity Clusters in Autism Spectrum Disorders: An Electronic Health Record Time-Series Analysis." *Pediatrics*, 133(1):54–63.

Dover, C. J., and Couteur A. Le. (2007). "How to Diagnose Autism." *Archives of Disease in Childhood*, 92 (6):540–45.

Dworzynski, K., A. Ronald, P. Bolton, and F. Happé. (2012). "How Different Are Girls and Boys Above and Below the Diagnostic Threshold for Autism Spectrum Disorders?" *Journal of the American Academy of Child Adolescent Psychiatry*, 51(8):788–97.

Elder, J. H., M. Shankar, J. Shuster, D. Theriaque, S. Burns, and L. Sherrill. (2006). "The Gluten-Free, Casein-Free Diet in Autism: Results of a Preliminary Double Blind Clinical Trial." *Journal of Autism and Developmental Disorders*, 36(3):413–20.

Granpeesheh, D., J. Tarbox, D. R. Dixon, A. E. Wilke, and M. S. Allen. (2010). "Bradstreet JJ. Randomized Trial of Hyperbaric Oxygen Therapy for Children with Autism." *Research in Autism Spectrum Disorders*, 4(2):268–75.

Green, D., S. Chandler, T. Charman, E. Simonoff, and G. Baird. (2016). "Brief Report: DSM-5 Sensory Behaviors in Children with and without an Autism Spectrum Disorder." *Journal of Autism and Developmental Disorders*, 46(11):3597–606.

Horvath, K., and J. A. Perman. (2002). "Autism and Gastrointestinal Symptoms." *Current Gastroenterology Reports,* 4(3):251–8.

Hens, K. (2019). "The Many Meanings of Autism: Conceptual and Ethical Reflections." *Development of Medical Child Neurology*, 61(4):1025–1029.

Hertz-Picciotto, I., R. J. Schmidt, and P. Krakowiak. (2018). "Understanding Environmental Contributions to Autism: Causal Concepts and the State of Science." *Autism Research*, 11(2): 554–586.

Inamdar, N. R., and N. Parajpe, N. (1981). "Administration of Social Welfare Programs for Physically Handicapped in India." *The Indian Journal of Public Administration,* xxvii (93):568–577.

Johnson, C. P., and S. M. Myers. (2007). "Identification and Evaluation of Children with Autism Spectrum Disorders." *Pediatrics*, 120 (5):1183–215.

Kern, J. K., V. S. Miller, L. Cauller, R. Kendall, J. Mehta, and M. Dodd. (2001). "Effectiveness of N, N-Dimethylglycine in Autism and Pervasive Developmental Disorder." *Journal of Child Neurology*, 16(3):169–73.

Kim, J., T. Wigram, and C. Gold. (2009). "Emotional, Motivational and Interpersonal Responsiveness of Children with Autism in Improvisational Music Therapy." *Autism*, 13(4):389–409.

King, B. H., N. Navot, R. Bernier, and S. J. Webb. (2014). "Update on Diagnostic Classification in Autism." *Current Opinion in Psychiatry*, 27(2):105–17.

Kolevzon, A., L. Bush, A. T. Wang, D. Halpern, Y. Frank, D. Grodberg, R. Rapaport, T. Tavassoli, W. Chaplin, L. Soorya, and J. D. Buxbaum. (2014). "A Pilot Controlled Trial of Insulin-Like Growth Factor-1 in Children with Phelan-McDermid Syndrome." *Molecular Autism*, 5(1):1–9.

Kossyvaki, L., and D. Papoudi. (2016). "A Review of Play Interventions for Children with Autism at School." *International Journal of Disability, Development, and Education*. 63(1):45–63.

Kuriyama, S., M. Kamiyama, M. Watanabe, S. Tamahashi, I. Muraguchi, T. Watanabe, A. Hozawa, T. Ohkubo, Y. Nishino, Y. Tsubono, and I. Tsuji. (2002). "Pyridoxine Treatment in a Subgroup of Children with Pervasive Developmental Disorders." *Developmental Medicine and Child Neurology*, 44(4):283–6

Lord, C., T. S. Brugha, T. Charman, J. Cusack, G. Dumas, T. Frazier, E. J. Jones, R. M. Jones, and A. Pickles. (2020). "Autism Spectrum Disorder." *Nature Reviews Disease Primers*, 6(1):1–23.

Loomes, R., L. Hull, and W. P. Mandy. (2017). "What Is the Male-to-Female Ratio in Autism Spectrum Disorder? A Systematic Review and Meta-Analysis." *Journal of the American Academy of Child and Adolescent Psychiatry*, 56(6):466–74.

Maestro, S., F. Muratori, M. C. Cavallaro, F. Pei, D. Stern, B. Golse, and F. Palacio-Espasa. (2002). "Attentional Skills during the First Six Months of Age in Autism Spectrum Disorder." *Journal of the American Academy of Child and Adolescent Psychiatry*, 41(10):1239–1245.

Myers, S. M., and C. P. Johnson. (2007). "Management of Children with Autism Spectrum Disorders." *Pediatrics,* 120(5):1162–82.

Navarro-Pardo, E., F. López-Ramón, Y. Alonso-Esteban, and F. Alcantud-Marín. (2021). "Diagnostic Tools for Autism Spectrum Disorders by Gender: Analysis of Current Status and Future Lines." *Children*, 8 (4):262–271.

Owen, R., L. Sikich, R. N. Marcus, P. Corey-Lisle, G. Manos, R. D. McQuade, W. H. Carson, and R. L. Findling. (2009). "Aripiprazole in the Teatment of Irritability in Children and Adolescents with Autistic Disorder." *Pediatrics*, 124(6):1533–40.

Ozonoff, S., G. S. Young, J. Brian, T. Charman, E. Shephard, A. Solish, and L. Zwaigenbaum. (2018). "Diagnosis of Autism Spectrum Disorder after Age Five in Children Evaluated Longitudinally since Infancy." *Journal of the American Academy of Child and Adolescent Psychiatry*, 57(11):849–57.

Paavonen, E. J., W. T. Nieminen-von, R. Vanhala, E. T. Aronen, and L. von Wendt. (2003). "Effectiveness of Melatonin in the Treatment of Sleep Disturbances in Children with Asperger Disorder." *Journal of Child Adolescent Psychopharmacol*, 13(1):83–95.

Pandey, J., A. Verbalis, D. L. Robins, H. Boorstein, A. M. Klin, T. Babitz, K. Chawarska, F. Volkmar, J. Green, M. Barton, and D. Fein. (2008). "Screening for Autism in Older and Younger Toddlers with the Modified Checklist for Autism in Toddlers." *Autism*, 12(5):513–35.

Penner, M., E. Anagnostou, L. Y. Andoni, and W. J. Ungar. (2018). "Systematic Review of Clinical Guidance Documents for Autism Spectrum Disorder Diagnostic Assessment in Select Regions." *Autism*, 22(5):517–527.

Plioplys, A. V. (1998). "Intravenous Immunoglobulin Treatment of Children with Autism." *Journal of Child Neurology*, 13(2):79–82.

Politi, P., H. Cena, M. Comelli, G. Marrone, C. Allegri, E. Emanuele, and S. U. di Nemi. (2008). "Behavioral Effects of Omega-3 Fatty Acid Supplementation in Young Adults with Severe Autism: An Open-Label Study." *Archives of Medical Research*, 39(7):682–5.

Reichow, B., E. E. Barton, B. A. Boyd, and K. Hume. (2012). Early Intensive Behavioral Intervention (EIBI) for Young Children with Autism Spectrum Disorder (ASD). Cochrane Database of Systematic Reviews, 122(10): 23–30.

Robins, D. L. (2008). "Screening for Autism Spectrum Disorders in Primary Care Settings." *Autism*, 12(5):537–56.

Robins, D. L., D. Fein, and M. Barton. (2009). "The Modified Checklist for Autism in Toddlers, Revised with Follow-up." *Pediatrics*, 133(3):37–45.

Rogers, S. J., A. Estes, C. Lord, J. Munson, M. Rocha, J. Winter, J. Greenson, C. Colombo, G. Dawson, L. A. Vismara, and C. A. Sugar. (2019). "A Multisite Randomized Controlled Two-Phase Trial of the Early Start Denver Model Compared to Treatment as Usual." *Journal of the American Academy of Child and Adolescent Psychiatry*, 58(9): 853–65.

Rudenstine, S., and S. Galea. (2015). "Preventing Brain Disorders: A Framework for Action." *Social Psychiatry and Psychiatric Epidemiology*, 50(4): 833–841.

Sarker, Profulla C. (2017). *Sociocultural Parameters of Health and Diseases*. Dhaka: Mother's Publications

Sanchack, K., and C. A. Thomas. (2016). "Autism Spectrum Disorder: Primary Care Principles." *American Family Physician*, 94(12):972–9.

Schneider, C. K., R. D. Melmed, L.E. Barstow, F. J. Enriquez, J. Ranger-Moore, and J. A. Ostrem. (2006). "Oral Human Immunoglobulin for Children with Autism and Gastrointestinal Dysfunction: A Prospective, Open-Label Study." *Journal of Autism and Developmental Disorders*, 36(8):1053–64.

Shaw, K. A., M. J. Maenner, and J. Baio, (2020). "Early Identification of Autism Spectrum Disorder among Children Aged Four Years-Early Autism and Developmental Disabilities Monitoring Network, Six Sites, United States." *MMWR Surveill Summ*, 69(3):1–12.

Shivers, C. M., and J. B. Plavnick. (2015). "Sibling Involvement in Interventions for Individuals with Autism Spectrum Disorders: A Systematic Review". *Journal of Autism Development Disord*, 45(3):685–96.

Taylor, W. W., and I. W. Taylor. (1970). *Services for the Handicapped in India*. New York: International Society for Handicapped of the Disabled.

Vahdatpour, C., A. H. Dyer, and D. Tropea. (2016). "Insulin-Like Growth Factor 1 and Related Compounds in the Treatment of Childhood-Onset Neurodevelopmental Disorders." *Frontiers in Neuroscience*, 10 (2):450.

Waldman, Peter E. (1982). "The Rehabilitation of Disabled People: Toward a Framework for Future Development." *International Journal of Rehabilitation Research*, 12(3):317–325.

Werling, D. M., and D. H. Geschwind. (2013). "Understanding Sex Bias in Autism Spectrum Disorder." *Proceedings of the National Academy of Sciences of the United States of America*, 110(13):4868–9.

Whitehouse, A. J., J. Granich, G. Alvares, M. Busacca, M. N. Cooper, A. Dass, T. Duong, R. Harper, W. Marshall, A. Richdale, and T. Rodwell. (2017). "A Randomised Controlled Trial of an IP Ad-Based Application to Complement Early Behavioral Intervention in Autism Spectrum Disorder." *Journal of Child Psychology and Psychiatry,* 58(9):1042–52.

Yates, K., and Couteur A. Le. (2016). "Diagnosing Autism Spectrum Disorders." *Journal of Paediatrics and Child Health,* 26(12):513–8.

Yirmiya, N., and T. Charman. (2010). "The Prodrome of Autism: Early Behavioral and Biological Signs, Regression, Peri- and Post-Natal Development and Genetics." *Journal of Child Psychology and Psychiatry,* 51(4):432–58.

Zwaigenbaum, L., and M. Penner. (2018). "Autism Spectrum Disorder: Advances in Diagnosis and Evaluation." *BMJ.* 6 (2). 361–379.

Chapter 13

COUNSELING AGAINST CONSANGUINITY FOR INBRED COMMUNITY

Introduction

Consanguineous marriages are preferred and allowed to be practiced among Muslims in Bangladesh. Many people do not know the consequences of consanguinity on the health-related problems of offspring. Studies revealed that most people are unaware of the consequences of consanguinity on the etiology of diseases for the next generations (Imaizumi 1986). In Bangladesh, very few studies have been conducted to determine the current prevalence of consanguinity and its effects on genetic disorders like autism in the offspring. Autism is a lifelong developmental disability that affects how people perceive, communicate, and interact with others. However, it is essential to recognize that there are differing opinions on this, and not all autistic people are considered disabled. This chapter emphasizes the causative factor in raising the incidence of genetic diseases, especially autism, of the offspring of two hundred parents whose marriages were confined to cross-cousin and parallel cousins. The adverse effects of autism are found among the progeny due to the genes received from common ancestors. Marriages were classified according to the degree of the relationship between couples, including cross-cousin and parallel cousin, which may be either patrilineal or matrilineal. Before the Autism Act in Bangladesh, autism was often misunderstood by the general people and professionals. As a result, too many autistic people face significant barriers to living whole and rewarding lives in the community. Action should be taken to improve services and support for autistic people and their families to improve society's awareness about autism in Bangladesh.

Despite the advancement of medical science, healthcare facilities, increasing literacy, expansion of urbanization, and employment opportunities, the family-linked traditions are yet to be broken. In recent times, the situation appears better in urban areas. In a population with a high degree of inbreeding, the formulation of a public health program with a multi-approach strategy, including educating the people about the anticipated genetic consequences upon the offspring, prenatal diagnosis, neonatal screening, and genetic counseling is essential in a community where consanguineous marriages are prevailing.

Concept of Genetic Counseling

It is not easy to develop a uniform definition of genetic counseling. It consists of those biocultural practices, methods, techniques, and substances embedded in a matrix of values, traditions, beliefs, and patterns of ecological and genetic adaptation that provide the means for maintaining genetic health and preventing or ameliorating genetic disorder of the offspring of the parents, especially those involved in consanguineous marriage (Press 1980).

Genetic counseling is the process of awareness that is given to the prospective brides and grooms, along with their parents or guardians, for the selection of life partners to avoid genetic disorders in their offspring. Even awareness counseling needs to be given to newly wedded couples who are already married among their relatives for prenatal screening to avoid genetic disorders in their offspring. Usually, genetic counseling is given to the targeted couples who might be the future parents about the consequences and nature of the disorder, the probabilities of developing, and the choices open to them in the management and planning of their families to prevent, avoid, or ameliorate the disorder upon their offspring. This has preventive, diagnostic, therapeutic, and supportive value. Genetic counseling is considered to prevent the adverse effects of the shared genes on offspring that are inherited through the consanguineous marriages of the parents.

Genetic counseling is also considered an essential part of the management of patients and families in which a genetic disorder has been diagnosed or who are at risk for such a disease. It gives patients the necessary information about the disease and their genetic profile. Also, it calculates the risk or probability of a genetic disorder appearing in their family and provides support, diagnosis, and management facilities and treatment. Most of the people of Bangladesh need to be made aware of the inheritance patterns and risk factors of genetic diseases, which pose additional challenges to their implementation of genetic services. Thus, along with developing infrastructure for genetic service delivery, comprehensive public awareness programs should be introduced throughout the country to provide knowledge on the deleterious effects and possible preventive measures of genetic diseases and the role of consanguinity as one of the causes. Moreover, suitable measures need to be taken to ensure proper treatment and follow-up for patients with genetic diseases like autism. However, autism is not a disease. Instead, it is considered a developmental disorder.

Genetic Counseling in Bangladesh

With the advancement of genetic and genomic science and public health care services in the twenty-first century, genetic counseling services have become an integral part of medical science worldwide, especially where consanguineous marriages are encouraged and practiced. It is revealed in different studies that consanguinity is significantly high in Muslim countries because consanguineous marriages are allowed in Islamic culture. It is also found that reproductive diseases are associated with genetic disorders due to gene mutation with the same genetic pole due to inbreeding. It has been observed that many children are affected by different gene-related diseases of inbred communities due to consanguinity. Many people are not aware of the effect of consanguinity upon children due to poor knowledge about the impact of consanguineous marriages. Under the circumstances, they need to be aware to avoid consanguineous marriages. At the same time, they require genetic counseling services to prevent genetic disorders in children, and services should be given to those who are already affected by genetic disorders like autism. Consequently, genetic disorders are emerging as a significant public health concern in many countries, including Bangladesh, where consanguineous marriages are preferred.

Inherited inborn disorders of children have been identified globally, and common genetic diseases are increasingly emerging as a significant health challenge (Morton 1978; Lewis, R. 2009). Early and accurate diagnosis of these diseases is critical to optimal patient care. However, diagnosing genetic diseases can be challenging and contingent upon understanding the disease's molecular etiology. Although understanding many human diseases has advanced significantly in the post-genomic era, studies revealed that the knowledge of most genetic diseases is still meager. Moreover, the treatment of diseases due to genetic disorders is costly. Some of the parents of autistic children have already reported that the scope of treatment of their autistic children is minimal and is concentrated in urban settings of Bangladesh and, at the same time, lengthy process of treatment. Under the circumstances, it is difficult for the parents of autistic children to stay in the urban setting for a long time for the treatment of their children. Even autistic children have minimal scope for schooling for special education. It is challenging for parents to treat diseases related to genetic disorders in their offspring. The expertise, infrastructure, and expenses required for genetic disease treatment are not limited to Bangladesh. Moreover, these facilities are polarized to urban settings, which are already mentioned elsewhere in this chapter. It should be noted that there is a dearth of knowledge of genetic diseases among medical graduates in Bangladesh. In addition, inadequate psychosocial support, religious values, and sociocultural stigma often influence the treatment of the patients of genetic disorders for autistic children.

Process of Genetic Counselling

Genetic counseling is started in three phases, viz., the premarital phase of counseling, the prenatal phase through screening, and newborn screening, which covers the neonatal to infant phase. There is an individual process for each phase. However, there is a network relationship among the different identified phases to provide genetic counseling to reduce genetic disorders in children like autism. The following processes have been explained to get a clear idea of how genetic counseling takes place.

- **Premarital Counseling:** Premarital counseling is considered the first step to minimizing genetic disease transmission from parents to their offspring (Saf and Howard 2015). It is imperative to reduce the transmission of autosomal recessive disorders in the context of consanguineous marriages, the genetic burden of which Bangladeshis do not usually comprehend properly (El-Hazmi 2004). Awareness campaigns are likely to contribute a significant part to the success of premarital counseling. This counseling has become popular in the Middle East, where consanguineous marriages are widely practiced. Similar programs have already been implemented in Italy, Iran, and Greece, achieving significant results. Consequently, premarital counseling is regarded as one of the most effective measures to reduce the incidence of genetic diseases associated with a high carrier frequency in the offspring.

- **Prenatal Screening:** Premarital screening could be followed by prenatal screening as the second step for early diagnosis of congenital abnormalities (Gregg et al., 2013). The scope of the prenatal screening system is unavailable in many countries, including Bangladesh. An important reason for the lack of prenatal screening is the technical inability of most of the hospitals in developing countries to perform confirmatory molecular or genetic tests for chromosomal abnormalities (e.g., Down syndrome). In many cases, diagnosis mainly depends on the general clinical features. It should be taken into account that while most pregnancies in city areas are often followed carefully, perhaps by using modern ultra-sonography techniques, this is only a rare case in rural areas of Bangladesh, where one-fourth of the people live (Hamamy 2012).

- **Neonatal Screening:** Newborn screening, finally, is a simple test at birth that can identify genetic conditions that may affect a child's long-term health or survival but are treatable at birth (DeSouza et al. 2019). In many countries, newborn screening programs have dramatically improved the morbidity and mortality associated with the disorders screened (Schulpen et al., 2006). However, in many other countries, mainly developing countries, including Bangladesh, Newborn Screening (NBS) programs are not as successful because of the diagnostic accuracy but for sociocultural and health-education-related reasons. Indeed, successful implementation of NBS requires a comprehensive system of education, follow-up, diagnosis, management, and evaluation that must be institutionalized and sustained within public health systems.

In most cases, implementing NBS programs is challenging for LICs and LMICs. In the last two decades, some LICs and LMICs in the Asia Pacific, Middle East, and North African regions initiated NBS; however, the progress is slow due to various factors, including poor economies, weak public health policies, and mediocre delivery methods (Tadmouri et al. 2009). Especially in the conservative cultural setup of the Indian subcontinent, like in Bangladesh, many people find clinical procedures as taboo-like phenomena and do not prefer to visit hospitals for labor purposes (Bennett et al. 2002; Bindu et al. 2006). Even those who decide to visit the hospital rarely allow sampling by invasive techniques (e.g., blood collected by heel pricking of the newborn). As a result, collecting samples from newborns is challenging (Cambell 2006). In some specific regions of Bangladesh, the Government tried to run a pilot project for NBS, especially for congenital hypothyroidism, but no nationwide institutionalized and sustainable NBS program is currently available (Nalini et al. 2008; Dousset 2018).

Role of Genetic Counselor

As healthcare team members, genetic counselors act as patient advocates, protecting their best interests and working as a genetic resource to physicians. Genetic counselors provide helpful information and support to families at risk of an array of inherited disorders. They are involved in identifying families at risk, investigating problems presented by the family, interpreting information about the disorder, analyzing inheritance patterns, and evaluating recurrence risks while reviewing testing options available to the family (Levitt, 2003). When autism is identified in a child of a consanguineous couple, investigations and referrals must proceed systematically, as clinically indicated for the presenting symptoms, but with an emphasis on autosomal recessive conditions in the diagnosis. Nevertheless, it is essential to remember that autosomal recessive conditions can arise by chance, with the child having two different mutations, not necessarily because of consanguineous marriage alone. This can go a long way in eliminating shame and guilt in the parents, that, somehow, they were responsible for the condition of their child, or in erasing the misconception that God is punishing them for their sin of marrying within the close family (Levitt 2003; Hussain 1998).).

Apart from autosomal recessive conditions leading to learning difficulties, consanguinity has not always been reported to have any significant effect on autism. A family history of possible autosomal recessive condition may considerably increase the risk of offspring over the background risks of consanguinity. The consanguineous couples can be tested for their carrier status and prenatal diagnosis when necessary. Investigating an affected relative may provide valuable clues when the diagnosis or mutation is unknown. If this is not possible, an estimation of the risks involved and detailed, systematic fetal scans are the only options open. However, this may leave many couples disconcerted by the residual uncertainty (Heidari et al. 2014; Dousset 2018).

Genetic counselors motivate the young generations and their parents before selecting a bride and groom for the marriage. If they choose their life partners within the kinship relations considering the socioeconomic quasi-economic interest of both parties, then there is a probability of autism in their offspring. Under the circumstances, the main slogan of the genetic counselors to the young generation and their parents is that the selection of bride or groom should not be by chance but somewhat by choice considering the fate of the future generations.

Tips in Counseling against Consanguinity

The young age of marriage in consanguineous couples further implicates a need to increase awareness programs among the young generation about the deleterious effects of consanguineous marriages. Such marriages' sociocultural and economic benefits are paramount to consanguineous couples and their relatives. However, the availability of preventive measures should be emphasized. Further, a genetic investigation is required to elucidate the mode of inheritance in this area. The following tips are identified to avoid autism.

- Refer well before conception, especially if they have a family history of a possible autosomal recessive condition.
- Remember to empathize and not imply that a child's condition is the parents' fault, even if the couples are consanguineous and the child has two identical copies of a mutant gene. Nobody deliberately passes on an illness to their offspring, and no one is to blame.
- Ensure the couple referred for premarital genetic counseling is informed that no blood tests provide General Genetic Compatibility data. They must be advised that some basic carrier tests are available for a limited range of specific conditions.
- Adopt a nonjudgmental attitude and a positive mindset to disseminate knowledge and information to the couple, empowering them with the various options available and enabling them to make intelligent decisions.
- Deal with the issue in a sensitive, caring, and sensible manner.

Concluding Remarks

Genetic counseling is one of the essential techniques to prevent congenital diseases like autism. It plays an important and unique role in the decision-making process of autistic people in their different phases of life. Counseling autistic people contributes to their knowledge of how to survive in the competitive and globalized market economy through their efforts with complete confidence.

One basic principle in the health system is the priority of prevention to treatment, and the authorities need to provide practical and effective ways to reduce costs and provide equitable access to genetic counseling facilities. Indeed, the ethical process of these consultations will significantly impact couples' decision-making. Considering the statistics obtained in this study and the critical ethical issues, the following key points and recommendations may be considered:

- A comprehensive program that needs to be taken to prevent the birth of children with disabilities is a professional commitment in line with the principle of justice in the distribution of health resources.

- Consanguineous marriage is deeply rooted in the people's culture. As an initial step, a social awareness program about the disadvantages and consequences of consanguinity needs to be activated among the target group.

- Counselling should be initiated for the people of the inbred communities where consanguineous marriage is allowed, practiced, and even encouraged for socioeconomic interest to keep the property and renew the relationship in the kinship network.

- In Bangladesh, consanguineous marriage is allowed and practiced among the Muslims. To prevent genetic diseases like autism, a once-a-week counseling program needs to be initiated at the mosque by the priest.

References

Alswaidi, F. M., and S. J. O'Brien. (2009). "Premarital Screening Programs for Haemoglobinopathies, HIV and Hepatitis Viruses: Review and Factors Affecting Their Success." *Journal Medical Screening*, 16 (2):22–8.

Bennett, R., A. Motulsky, and A. Bittles. (2002). "Genetic Counseling and Screening of Consanguineous Couple and their Offspring: Recommendations of the National Society of Genetic Counselors." *Journal of Genetic Counseling*, (11): pp. 97–119.

Bindu, P. S., S. Desai, K. E. Shehanaz, M. Nethravathy, and P. K. Pal. (2006). "Clinical Heterogeneity in Hallervorden-Spatz Syndrome: A Clinicoradiological Study in Thirteen Patients from South India." *Brain Development*, (28):343–7.

Cambell, J. M. (2006). *Autism Spectrum Disorder*. In (Eds.) by R. W. Kamphaus and J. M. Cambell in Psycho-Diagnostic Assessment of Children. New Jersey: John Willey and Sons.

Cousens, N. E., C. L. Gaf, S. A. Metcalfe, and M. B. Delatycki. (2010). "Carrier Screening for β-thalassaemia: A Review of International Practice." *European Journal of Human Genetics*, 18 (4):1077–83.

DeSouza, A., V. Wolan, A. Battochio, S. Christian, S. Hume, and G. Johner. (2019). "Newborn Screening: Current Status in Alberta." Canada International Journal of Neonatal Screen, 12 (3):5:37.

Dousset, Laurent. (2018). *Australian Aboriginal Kinship: An Introductory Handbook with Particular Emphasis on the Western Desert*. Manuels du Credo, Marseille: Pacific-credo Publications.

El-Hazmi, M. A. F. (2004). "The Natural History and the National Premarital Screening Program in Saudi Arabia." *Saudi Medical Journal*, 25 (4):1549–54.

Gregg, A. R., S. J. Gross, R. G. Best, K. G. Monaghan, K. Bajaj, and B. G. Skotko. (2013). "ACMG Statement on Noninvasive Prenatal Screening for Fetal Aneuploidy." *Genetic Medicine*, 15 (3):395–8.

Hamamy, Hanan (2012). "Consanguineous Marriage Perception Consultation in Primary Health Care Settings." *Journal of Community Genetics*, 3(3): 185–192.

Heidari, F., S. Dastgiri, and N. Tajaddini. (2014). "Prevalence and Risk Factors of Consanguineous Marriage." *European Journal of General Medicine* [serial online]. 11(4):248–255.

Hussain, R. (1998). "The Impact of Consanguinity and Inbreeding on Perinatal Mortality in Karachi, Pakistan." *Pediatric and Perinatal Epidemiology*, (12): pp. 370–382.

Imaizumi, Y. (1986). "A Recent Survey of Consanguineous Marriages in Japan." *Clinical Genetics*, 30 (3): 230–233.

Kanner, L. (1943). "Autism Disturbances of Affective Contact." *Nervous Child*, 4 (2): 217–250.

Karimi, M., N. Jamalian, H. Yarmohammadi, A. Askarnejad, A. Afrasiabi, and Hashemi. (2007). "Premarital Screening for β-thalassemia in Southern Iran: Options for Improving the Program." *Journal of Medical Screen*, 14 (2):62–6.

Levitt, G. (2003). Incest/inbreeding taboos. *International Encyclopedia of Marriage and Family*. Available at: http:// family.jrnk.org/pges/854/incest-inbreeding-Taboos-Sibling-Marriage-Human-Isolates.himil. Accessed March 28, 2015.

Lewis, R. (2009). *Human Genetics: Concepts and Applications*. New York: McGraw-Hill.

McWhirter, R. E., R. McQuillan, E. Visser, C. Counsell, and J. F. Wilson. (2012). "Genome-Wide Homozygosity and Multiple Sclerosis in Orkney and Shetland Islanders." *European Journal of Human Genetics*, 20(2), 198–202.

Morton, N. E. (1978). "Effect of Inbreeding on IQ and Mental Retardation." *Proceedings of National Academy of Sciences USA*, 75(8): 3906–3908.

Nalini, A., N. Gayathri, Yasha, T.C., Ravishankar, S., Urtizberea, A., and Huehne, K. (2008). "Clinical, Pathological and Molecular Findings in two Siblings with Giant Axonal Neuropathy (GAN): Report from India." *Eur J. Med Genet* (51):426-35.

Press, Irwin (1980). "Problems in the Definition and Classification of Medical System." Social Science and Medicine, 14B (1):45-57.

Saf, M. and Howard, N. (2015). "Exploring the effectiveness of Mandatory Premarital Screening and Genetic Counseling programs for β-thalassaemia in the Middle East: A Scoping Review." *Public Health Genomics*, 18 (3):193–203.

Schulpen, T. W., J. C. Wieringen, P. J. Brummen, J. M. Riel, F. A. Beemer, P. Westers, and J. Huber. (2006). "Infant Mortality, Ethnicity, and Genetically Determined Disorders in the Netherlands." *European Journal of Public Health*, 16 (1):291–294.

Tadmouri, G. O., P. Nair, T. Obeid, M. T. Al Ali, N. Al Khaja, and H. A. Hamamy. (2009). "Consanguinity and Reproductive Health among Arabs." *Reproductive Health*, 8 (6):17–23.

Chapter 14

TRAINING FOR PARENTS OF CHILDREN WITH AUTISM SPECTRUM DISORDER

Introduction

Since the 1960s, parents' training for autism spectrum disorder (ASD) in their offspring, referred to as parent education, has been developed and tested for a variety of childhood problems and disruptive behavior disorders (DBD) of autistic children (Eyberg et al. 2008). The main objective of this training was to educate the parents to enhance their parenting skills to capacity and competence to reduce specific childhood behavior problems of autistic children. The parents' training focuses on the triple *P,* indicating that the Positive Parenting Program (PPP) established criteria for evidence-based practices in treating these disorders (Eyberg et al. 2008). This chapter on parents' training is particularly relevant to developing the capacity of the parents to socialize with their children who are victims of autism spectrum disorder (ASD). Parenting interventions for disruptive behavior development (DBD) of autistic children are rooted in the mindset of parents conditioning some procedures through educating them in intensive training. In the 1960s, researchers explored and began using these procedures to reduce disruptive behaviors and encourage prosocial development in children with ASD (Ferster 1961; Ferster and Simons 1966; Patterson and Brodsky 1966). The main focus of this chapter is to explain to what extent different methods and techniques are used for parent training to reduce the problems of autism spectrum disorder (ASD).

Discrete Trial Training for the Parents

There is a growing interest in examining the impact of parents implementing Discrete Trial Training (DTT). One of the earliest studies examined the parent's involvement in Discrete Trial Training (Lovaas et al. 1973), which demonstrated the importance of parents as agents of change in extending and maintaining the behavioral gains made by their children during the intervention. Subsequent studies have also illustrated that parent Discrete Trial Training (DTT) programs can effectively teach sophisticated behavioral procedures and concepts that are prompting, fading, shaping, chaining, reinforcement, punishment, data collection, generalization, and maintenance in working with children with autism (Anderson et al. 1987; Harris 1983; Koegel et al. 1978; Smith et al. 2000). At the same time, numerous studies have demonstrated the parent's ability to acquire the skills necessary to teach their children and generalization, or the parents' skill level in transferring their child's learning objectives to other behaviors. It has been noted as a weakness in this parent's training intervention approach (Baker 1989; Koegel et al. 1978).

Crockett et al. (2007) recently examined parents' implementation of DTT procedures to enhance the generalization of untrained child skills and cost-effectiveness. The primary investigation demonstrated control of the training program over parents' correct use of DTT and generalized effects of training on multiple functional child skills. While such results are encouraging, systematic replications with more participants are needed to strengthen and build upon training procedures to enhance generalization. The teaching practices of DTT emphasize the importance of a structured and adult-guided learning environment in the early stages of teaching children with autism (Smith et al. 2001). However, an essential goal for behavioral PT programs is to equip parents with an effective way of teaching their children the many skills they need to live optimally in their daily environments. Within this general framework, there has been a search for intervention approaches that can produce generalized improvements and target core areas that may impact many broad areas of functioning. Behavioral PT approaches encompass more naturalistic teaching procedures that may help address this requirement.

Significance of Training for the Parents

The target learners in parent training intervention are typically the child's primary caregivers. This may include a child's mother, father, grandparents, or other interested family members. Studies revealed that most of the participants in parent training were mothers. However, there is growing research on how to involve fathers along with other caregivers of autistic children in training programs (Seung et al. 2006). Parents' participation is probably more critical because they are motivated and committed to learning new skills (Kaiser and Hancock, 2003). Further, at least one parent must attend all sessions to increase consistency and facilitate learning. Parent stress is another important consideration when determining who should participate in a parent training program. Research demonstrates reductions in child-related stress following this training program (Moes 1995). Studies have also documented that parents who are experiencing clinical levels of parent-related stress, including depression, marital discord, or health issues, do not benefit as much as parents who do not demonstrate clinically elevated stress (Robbins et al. 1991). The main topics of significance of parents' training are the following:

- **Efficiency of Services:** Studies revealed the importance of parent training in increasing the quantity and availability of intervention while requiring less time for child gains than clinician-implemented intervention (Koegel et al. 1982). Recent research on intensive short-term parent training demonstrates that once parents are trained to deliver intervention strategies to their autistic children, they can effectively train other family members and service providers (Symon 2005). Consequently, the services to the targeted autistic children become accessible at the family level in the kinship network system and thus contribute to reducing the many problems of autistic children in their daily functioning (McClanahan et al. 1982).

- **Implementation of Behavioral Intervention:** Research has demonstrated that the trained parents of children with ASD can effectively implement behavioral intervention strategies with a high degree of fidelity (Koegel et al. 2002; Koegel et al. 1996; Laski et al. 1988). They learned to use techniques that lead to reductions in problem behaviors (Frea and Hepburn 1999; Sofronoff et al. 2004) through increased child functional communication skills, increased child joint attention skills, developed play skills, improved social skills, and reduced sleeping problems (Rocha et al. 2007; Stahmer 1995; Weiskop et al. 2005).

- **Increased Parent-Child Interactions:** In addition to expanding the skills acquired by children and parents' delivery of specific intervention strategies, numerous other positive effects on the family have been documented in the following parent training programs. Early ASD parent training research documented positive impacts on parent-child interactions. For example, in a study comparing the effects of parent versus clinician-implemented intervention. Koegel et al. (1992) found that children who received parent training intervention responded more to their parents' questions and directions. Likewise, parents of children with ASD have demonstrated increased positive affect (Koegel et al. 1996; Schreibman et al. 1991), reduced stress (Moes 1995), and reported more time for leisure activities (Koegel et al. 1984).

- **Improvement of Spontaneous Vocalizations:** Children showed improvements in the number of spontaneous vocalizations, imitative behaviors, and overall engagement and initiations during interactions with their parents and with therapists in weekly sessions. During any phase of this study, children were not observed to exhibit high rates of problem behavior, such as screaming, throwing, biting, or noncompliance. The low level of disruptive behaviors may have been prevented by the use of motivational components, i.e., reinforcing child attempts, child-preferred activities, stimulus variation, and direct response reinforcer relationships within naturalistic play routines, as indicated by prior research (Dunlap and Koegel 1980; Koegel and Williams 1980).

- **Optimism toward Child's Future Increased**: Parents can evaluate their children's primary outcome progress through parent's training program. Evaluation of therapist progress notes indicates that 90 percent of the home-based practice assignments were implemented. For example, homework was done, and parents followed the reward systems. Studies revealed that 80 percent of the weekly home-based assignments were completed correctly and consistently when examining the quality of the home-based practice assignments. Other studies also revealed that parents' satisfaction with building confidence was finally assessed and found satisfactory. Parents reported a high level of satisfaction with the program, endorsing feeling *very satisfied* with the quality of the treatment and their child's progress, that their child was *improved* or *much improved*, and that their optimism toward their child's future increased.

- **Positive Treatment Response of the Children:** In terms of anxiety outcomes, results of the different research reports indicate that 92.9 percent of the treatment completers in the immediate treatment condition met the criteria for positive treatment response, compared to only 9.1 percent of the children whose parents did not participate in parent training. It is found that in parenting training, children with autism get full-time learning support from the parents and other family members using the trainers' instruction followed by the training module and thus stimulates the targeted autistic children to be socialized to lead an everyday life like their children.

Methods of Training for the Parents

There are three main methods used for training parents whose children are autistic. These methods are (1) naturalistic behavior methods, (2) integrated developmental and behavioral, and (3) cognitive behavioral methods. All these methods have individual identities in providing training to educate the parents to take care of their autistic children. However, they are interconnected to each other in their application to get holistic results from the training.

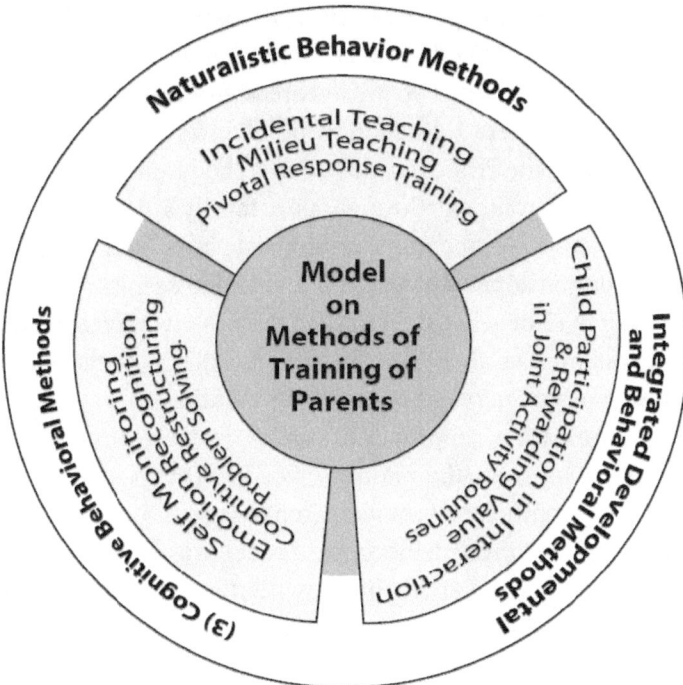

Fig. 8: Model on Methods of Training for Parents

- **Naturalistic Behavioral Methods:** The desire to improve the efficiency of behavioral interventions and response generalization leads to the development of less structured behavioral intervention methods that are provided in a natural context and involve intrinsically related rewards. There are multiple naturalistic behavioral methods, including incidental teaching (Hart and Risley 1968), milieu teaching (Hancock and Kaiser 2002), and, finally, pivotal response training (Koegel et al., 1987). This discussion focuses on pivotal response training, which was developed to target pivotal responses that result in widespread improvements in other nontargeted areas, representing an efficient method to produce generalized improvements (Koegel et al. 2003). This approach is a widely used intervention developed for parent training (National et al. 2001).

Many pivotal responses have been identified, which include child motivation, self-management, self-initiations, and responsivity to multiple cues (Koegel et al., 2001; Koegel et al., 1999; Schreibman and Koegel, 2005). However, most parent training research has focused on targeting two pivotal areas: motivation and responsivity to multiple cues. Intervention procedures targeting these areas are naturalistic strategies designed to be implemented in a child's natural environment throughout a family's daily routines using real-life, developmentally appropriate toys and materials. This intervention approach was first referred to as the natural language paradigm (Koegel et al. 1987) and later as pivotal response training (Schreibman et al. 1991). The PRT teaches parents to implement strategies to increase a child's motivation to engage in verbal communication, appropriate social interactions, and learning interactions from the natural environment (Koegel et al. 2003). Typically, clinicians provide parents with immediate and specific feedback on implementing the procedures described in written materials (Koegel et al., 1989) while the parent directly interacts with their child. These procedures include the (1) child's choice in the selection of toys and activities, (2) reinforcing apparent attempts, (3) interspersing maintenance with acquisition tasks, (4) responsivity to multiple cues, and (5) the use of contingent natural and direct reinforcers.

Naturalistic behavioral methods may be appropriate for a parents' training as they are intended to be incorporated more into an interaction style that a parent uses throughout the day, rather than a direct teaching method that may potentially burden a family by requiring a great deal of time to be set aside to teach individual target behaviors (Koegel and Koegel 2006; National et al. 2001; Wetherby and Wood, 2006). Attention should be given to developing the unique mental needs of young children and embedding teaching opportunities throughout meaningful daily activities and routines, pointing to the appropriateness of naturalistic behavior when addressing the needs of young children with autism (Koegel et al., 2008).

- **Integrated Behavioral Methods:** This section includes integrated developmental and behavioral methods. Behavioral interventions have been widely influential in addressing preschool and school-aged children's symptoms and learning needs (Levy et al., 2006). There is a pressing need to determine what type of changes or modifications in these intervention programs might be necessary to promote permanent and meaningful developmental growth in infants and toddlers (Boulware et al. 2006; Volkmar et al. 2005; Wetherby and Woods 2006), especially given the focus on early identification and diagnosis (Osterling et al. 2002). For example, researchers may need to adapt behavioral protocols to address specific developmental needs, such as the importance of teaching prelinguistic social communicative skills, e.g., joint attention and imitation, or to consider other realistic constraints, such as sleep schedules and feeding times.

The integration of developmental methods in behavioral intervention programs uses teaching strategies consistent with the principles of applied behavior analysis in treating the symptoms associated with ASD and concomitant delays; however, these approaches use typical developmental sequences as the content of their interventions and developmental theory as the guiding principle of their approach (Rogers and Ozonoff 2006). Like naturalistic behavioral programs, developmental approaches are child-directed in that teaching opportunities are arranged within the child's natural environment to elicit initiations. The adult then follows the child's lead by responding to the child's behavior and modeling, imitating, or expanding on the child's response. There is a strong focus on enhancing the child's relationship with others in the intervention, and as such, social engagement, reciprocity, and shared affect represent a significant priority of adult-child interactions. Additionally, these approaches emphasize the development of the full range of interpersonal communicative behaviors, including eye contact, shared affect, intentional vocalization, manual gestures, and speech, to achieve reciprocal communicative exchanges in interactions involving objects and social games. Although developmental interventions for ASD have not been studied as rigorously as behavioral treatments, empirical support is beginning to accumulate. A few published interventions exist, including two randomized controlled trials, which demonstrated efficacy with infants and toddlers at risk for

ASD (Mahoney et al.,1998; Mahoney and Perales, 2005; Strain and Hoyson, 2000).

There are a few integrated developmental and behavioral methods, including the Developmental Social Pragmatic (DSP) curriculum developed by Ingersoll and Dvortcsak (2006) and the Early Start Denver Model (ESDM), which focuses discussion on the ESDM, a manualized approach to parent training designed to precede intensive early intervention services for toddlers at risk for ASD, aged 12–36 months. The ESDM is a developmental, individualized, and relationship-based model to address the unique socio-emotional needs of infants and toddlers with ASD and their families. The three main goals of intervention in the ESDM are the following:

- Having the child participate in coordinated, interactive social interactions to build social attention, imitation, and symbolic communication skills.

- Increasing the child's reward value of social experiences with others by teaching within child-preferred activities and reading the child's cues and nonverbal behavior during play and

- Develop joint activity routines in which the child and partner co-construct and participate in play activities together so that the child can understand, predict, and complete the routine. At the same time, the adult "fills in" the learning deficits to build skills that include teaching, imitation, communication, flexible toy play, and awareness of social partners.

The ESDM curriculum draws extensively from two methods that have received empirical support for improving skill acquisition in children with ASD. The first approach, the Denver model developed by Rogers and colleagues, was shown to accelerate learning across various developmental domains (Rogers and DiLalla 1991; Rogers et al. 2001; Rogers et al. 1986; Rogers and Lewis 1989; Rogers et al. 1987). The Denver model focuses on building an effective, warm, and supportive environment to facilitate social engagement, reciprocity, and shared affect between children and adults. There is also a strong focus on approaching language development from a communication science orientation, addressing the social function of language, i.e., pragmatics and the development of nonverbal communication and imitation as the precursors to verbal language. The second model is pivotal response training, as described earlier.

- **Cognitive Behavioral Methods:** Incorporating parent training into interventions directed for school-age children and adolescents rather than toddlers and preschoolers with ASD and comorbid psychiatric disorders has been of increasing interest to researchers (Anderson and Morris 2006; Chalfant et al. 2007; Reaven and Hepburn 2003, 2006; Attwood and Hinton 2005; Sze and Wood 2007). A recent review of the trajectory of development in adolescents with ASD indicates that as children with ASD age, their symptoms of ASD, particularly communication deficits, may become less obvious to observers despite the continued pervasive impairments in their social skills and comprehension (Seltzer et al. 2004). Simultaneously, the prevalence of comorbid psychiatric diagnoses increases as children with ASD age (Simonoff et al. 2008). Internalizing disorders of anxiety and depression, for example, are common among children and adolescents with ASD, affecting 22–84 percent of the population (de Bruin et al. 2007; Ghaziuddin 1998; Green et al. 2000; Kim et al. 2000; Leyfer et al. 2006). The additional impairment in a child's social, family, and academic functioning associated with co-occurring psychiatric problems frequently merits intervention. Thus, as children with ASD age and associated psychiatric problems may emerge, the focus of interventions is to teach children strategies to cope with challenges that are commensurate with their cognitive and verbal abilities.

It is suggested that youth with a primary diagnosis of ASD and a comorbid diagnosis of anxiety or depression are likely to be incredibly responsive to learning cognitive coping strategies through interventions such as family cognitive-behavioral therapy (FCBT). This intervention model emphasizes teaching children and adolescents cognitive coping strategies such as self-monitoring, emotion identification and recognition, cognitive restructuring, and problem-solving. Through discussion and questioning, therapists and children identify maladaptive cognitions. The coping skills are learned early in treatment; tests of the "new" cognitions are planned and practiced in the treatment room and then gradually transferred into more naturalistic settings until the child can master the skill in the actual setting and across settings.

In vivo exposure involves implementing strategies practiced with the clinician but in real-life situations previously avoided, e.g., joining a game of tag on the playground. Exposures begin with conditions that are only slightly challenging and then, building on successes, increase in difficulty until mastery and generalization are evident. This is optimal for parents' involvement and training because in vivo exposures focus on gaining mastery outside the treatment room, where children would benefit most from developing their skills. Unlike traditional social and communication skills training and treatment of psychiatric disorders done in the treatment room, which rarely generalize to daily life, in vivo exposure techniques place training and practice in actual situations where generalization is desired through the involvement of parents, thus improving the chances of youth's spontaneous use of the skills in these environments after training is complete.

Parental involvement in these interventions has been found to enhance treatment effectiveness for typically developing children (Cobham et al. 1998; Mendlowitz et al. 1999), and emerging evidence suggests the same for children and adolescents with ASD (Reaven and Hepburn 2006; Sofronoff et al. 2005; Sze and Wood 2007). Parent involvement is essential for several reasons. First, child noncompliance with intervention goals may be inadvertently sustained by parents who are uncertain or inconsistent with efforts to manage and oversee their children's intervention adherence. As a result of the deficits in motivation associated with ASD, parents may provide unnecessary reassurance and assistance with feared situations, further promoting a sense of dependency in their children (Seligman 1972). Second, training parents to implement cognitive behavioral strategies outside the treatment room allows children to achieve mastery in varied settings with varied individuals, and treatment gains are likely to be maintained.

In the parent training component of this intervention, parents are provided with a rationale for targeting autonomy-supporting behaviors and communication skills by emphasizing the importance of these skills in their child's adaptive functioning and development into adulthood.

Parents are taught to support their children's attempts at courageous behavior, social skills, and independence through autonomy-supporting behaviors and communication skills. Autonomy-supporting behaviors include respecting the child's struggle; parents are trained to withhold assistance and provide their children time to figure out their solutions, allowing them to learn through trial and error. Additionally, communication skills, such as giving choices, are taught. Finally, parents are trained to provide immediate positive feedback or reinforcement to their children when reasonable attempts or mastery are made to increase their children's motivation to try again.

Role of Parent in Psychosocial Functioning

Although the role of parental factors is highly relevant to both the parents and their autistic children, it has been conceptualized differently in the development of PT intervention models for ASD and DBD. Parental stress and depression in parents of children with ASD have often been discussed as a result of raising a child with a disability (Moes 1995), while environmental stressors and parental psychopathology have been associated with increased child symptomatology in children with DBD. The results of the reviewed literature on current PT empirical research were consistent with these conceptual differences. ASD interventions were much more likely to explicitly state that parents are active collaborators in designing interventions for their children (Brookman-Frazee 2004) and address stress as a reaction to the child's issues and reductions in stress as an essential collateral effect of intervention (Koegel et al. 1996), while DBD interventions were more likely to explicitly target parent factors such as stress, depression, and marital problems as a structured part of their PT program that are suggestive of causal attributes to child issues (Kazdin and Whitley, 2003).

Concluding Remarks

Overall, this chapter suggests that parent training is a feasible and effective intervention method for children with ASD of varying ages and functioning levels (National et al. 2001). Many parents want to learn and be involved in their children's development. Because this approach is cost-efficient and increases the number of hours of teaching, many programs now include a parent training component (Koegel et al., 2008). Factors like marital discord, parental depression, severe child behavioral problems, and inadequate social support may interfere with families benefiting from traditional parent training (Stern 2000; Webster-Stratton and Reid 2003). Thus, researchers must continue to examine specific strategies and program components, e.g., directive vs. nondirective, to be incorporated into the parent training process that may be more effective for families who have not responded to traditional parent education approaches. Future studies concentrating on how best to integrate concrete behavioral procedures while emphasizing parental empowerment and family support will be especially critical for parents of children with autism. In the area of community practice, additional research is needed to address how to implement research-based parent training interventions most effectively in 'usual care' community settings, such as how to train community-based providers most efficiently and how to reach families that may be less motivated than those who participate in university-based intervention studies.

References

Anderson, S., and J. Morris. (2006). "Cognitive Behavior Therapy for People with Asperger Syndrome." *Behavioral and Cognitive Psychotherapy,* 34(2): 293–303.

Anderson, S. R., D. L., Avery, E. K., DiPietro, G. L. Edwards, and W. P. Christian. (1987). "Intensive Home-Based Early Intervention with Autistic Children." *Education and Treatment of Children,* 10 (4): 352–366.

Baker, B. L. (1989). *Parent Training and Developmental Disabilities.* Washington: American Association on Mental Retardation.

Boulware, G., I. S. Schwartz, S. R. Sandall, and B. J. McBride. (2006). "Project DATA for Toddlers: An Inclusive Approach to Very Young Children with Autism Spectrum Disorder." *Topics in Early Childhood Special Education,* 26 (2): 94–105.

Brookman-Frazee, L. (2004). "Using Parent/Clinician Partnerships in Parent Education Programs for Children with Autism." *Journal of Positive Behavior Interventions,* 6 (2): 195–213.

Cobham, V. E., M. R. Dadds, and S. H. Spence. (1998). "The Role of Parental Anxiety in the Treatment of Childhood Anxiety." *Journal of Consulting and Clinical Psychology,* 66 (4): 893–905.

Chalfant, A. M., R., Rapee, and L. Carroll. (2007). "Treating Anxiety Disorders in Children with High-Functioning Autism Spectrum Disorders: A Controlled Trial." *Journal of Autism and Developmental Disorders,* 37(4): 1842–1857.

Crockett, J. L., R. K., Fleming, K. J., Doepke, and J. S. Stevens. (2007). "Parent Training: Acquisition and Generalization of Discrete Trials Teaching Skills with Parents of Children with Autism." *Research in Developmental Disabilities,* 28 (2): 23–36.

de Bruin, E. I., R. F. Ferdinand, S. Meester, P. F. A. de Nijs, and F. Verheij. (2007). "High Rates of Psychiatric Comorbidity in PDD-NOS." *Journal of Autism and Developmental Disorders*, 37(4): 877–886.

Dunlap, G., and R. L. Koegel. (1980). "Motivating Autistic Children through Stimulus Variation." *Journal of Applied Behavior Analysis*, 13, (3): 619–627.

Eyberg, S. M., M. M. Nelson, and S. R. Boggs. (2008). "Evidence-Based Psychosocial Treatments for Children and Adolescents with Disruptive Behavior." *Journal of Clinical Child and Adolescent Psychology*, 37 (3): 215–237.

Ferster, C. B. (1961). "Positive Reinforcement and Behavioral Deficits of Young Children." *Child Development*, 32 (4): 437–456.

Ferster, C. B., and J. Simons. (1966). "Behavior Therapy with Children." *Psychological Record*, 16 (2):65–71.

Frea, W. D., and S. L. Hepburn. (1999). "Teaching Parents of Children with Autism to Perform Functional Assessments to Plan Interventions for Extremely Disruptive Behaviors." *Journal of Positive Behavior Interventions*, 1(2): 112–116.

Ghaziuddin, M., E., Weidmer-Mikhail, and N. Ghaziuddin. (1998). "Comorbidity of Asperger Syndrome: A Preliminary Report." *Journal of Intellectual Disability Research*, 42(2): 279–283.

Green, J., A. Gilchrist, D. Burton, and A. Cox. (2000). "Social and Psychiatric Functioning in Adolescents with Asperger Syndrome Compared with Conduct Disorder." *Journal of Autism and Developmental Disorders*, 30(3):279–293.

Hancock, T. B., and A. P. Kaiser. (2002). "The Effects of Trainer-Implemented Enhanced Milieu Teaching on the Social Communication of Children with Autism." *Topics in Early Childhood Special Education*, 22 (3):39–54.

Harris, S. L. (1983). *Families of the Developmentally Disabled*. New York: Pergamon Press.

Hart, B. M., and T. R. Risley. (1968). "Establishing Use of Descriptive Adjectives in the Spontaneous Speech of Disadvantaged Preschool Children." *Journal of Applied Behavior Analysis*, 1(1):109–120.

Ingersoll, B., and A. Dvortcsak. (2006). "Including Parent Training in the Early Childhood Special Education Curriculum for Children with Autism Spectrum Disorders." *Journal of Positive Behavior Interventions*, 8(2) 79–87.

Kaiser, A. P., and T. B. Hancock. (2003). "Teaching Parents New Skills to Support their Young Children's Development." *Infants and Young Children*, pp. 16, 9–21.

Kazdin, A. E., and Whitley, M. K. (2003). "Treatment of Parental Stress to Enhance Therapeutic Change among Children Referred for Aggressive and Antisocial Behavior." *Journal of Consulting and Clinical Psychology*, 71 (4):504–515.

Kim, J. A., P. Szatmari, S. E. Bryson, D. L. Streiner, and F. J. Wilson. (2000). "The Prevalence of Anxiety and Mood Problems among Children with Autism and Asperger Syndrome." *Autism*, 4(2):117–132.

Koegel, R. L., A. Bimbela, and L. Schreibman. (1996). "Collateral Effects of Parent Training on Family Interactions." *Journal of Autism and Developmental Disorders*, 26 (3): 347–359.

Koegel, R. L., K. Dyer, and L. K. Bell. (1987). "The Influence of Child-Preferred Activities on Autistic Children's Social Behavior." *Journal of Applied Behavior Analysis*, 20 (3): 243–252.

Koegel, R. L., and L. K. Koegel. (2006). *Pivotal Response Treatments for Autism: Communication, Social, and Academic Development*. Baltimore: Paul H. Brookes Publishing Company.

Koegel, R. L., L. K. Koegel, and L. I. Brookman. (2003). "Empirically Supported Pivotal Response Interventions for Children with Autism." In A. E. Kazdin and J. R. Weisz (Eds.), *Evidence-Based Psychotherapies for Children and Adolescents.* New York: Guilford Press.

Koegel, L. K., R. L. Koegel, J. K. Harrower, and C. M. Carter. (1999). "Pivotal Response Intervention: Overview of Approach." *Journal of the Association for Persons with Severe Handicaps*, 24(2):174–185.

Koegel, R. L., L. K. Koegel, and E. K. McNerney. (2001). "Pivotal Areas in Intervention for Autism." *Journal of Clinical Child Psychology*, 30 (1): 19–32.

Koegel, L. K., R. L. Koegel, Y. Shoshan, and E. McNerney. (1999). "Pivotal Response Intervention II: Preliminary Long Term Outcome Data." *Journal of the Association for Persons with Severe Handicaps*, 24(3): 186–198.

Koegel, R. L., A. Bimbela, and L. Schreibman. (1996). "Collateral Effects of Parent Training on Family Interactions." *Journal of Autism and Developmental Disorders*, 26(4): 347–359.

Koegel, L. K., R. L. Koegel, R. M. Fredeen, and G. W. Gengoux. (2008). Naturalistic Behavioral Approaches to Treatment. In K. Chawarska, A. Klin and F. R. Volkmar (Eds.), Autism Spectrum Disorder in Infants and Toddlers: Diagnosis, Assessment, and Treatment. New York: Guilford Press.

Koegel, R. L., and L. K. Koegel. (2006). *Pivotal Response Treatments for Autism: Communication, Social, and Academic Development.* Baltimore: Paul H. Brookes Publishing Company.

Koegel, R. L., L. K. Koegel, and Surratt, A. (1992). "Language Intervention and Disruptive Behavior in Preschool Children with Autism." *Journal of Autism and Developmental Disorders*, 22(2):141–153.

Laski, K. E., M. H. Charlop, and L. Schreibman. (1988). "Training Parents to Use the Natural Language Paradigm to Increase their

Autistic Children's Speech." *Journal of Applied Behavior Analysis*, 21(2):391–400.

Levy, S., A. Kim, and M. L. Olive. (2006). "Interventions for Young Children with Autism: A Synthesis of the Literature." *Focus on Autism and Other Developmental Disabilities*, 21(1): 55–62.

Leyfer, O. T., S. E. Folstein, S. Bacalman, N. O. Davis, E. Dinh, and J. Morgan. (2006). "Comorbid Psychiatric Disorders in Children with Autism: Interview Development and Rates of Disorders." *Journal of Autism and Developmental Disorders*, 36 (4): 849–861.

Lovaas, O. I., R. Koegel, J. Q. Simmons, and J. S. Long. (1973). "Some Generalization and Follow-Up Measures on Autistic Children in Behavior Therapy." *Journal of Applied Behavior Analysis*, 6 (1):131–166.

Mahoney, G., G. Boyce, G. R. Fewell, D. Spiker, and C. A. Wheeden. (1998). "The Relationship of Parent-Child Interaction to the Effectiveness of Early Intervention Services for At-Risk Children and Children with Disabilities." *Topics in Early Childhood Special Education*, 18 (1):5–17.

Mahoney, G., and F. Perales. (2005). "The Impact of Relationship focused Intervention on Young Children with Autism Spectrum Disorders: A Comparative Study." *Journal of Developmental and Behavioral Pediatrics*, 26 (1):77–85.

McClannahan, L., P. Krantz, and G. McGee. (1982). "Parents as Therapists for Autistic Children: A Model for Effective Parent Training." *Analysis and Intervention in Developmental Disabilities*, 2(2): 223–252.

Mendlowitz, S. L., K. Manassis, S. Bradley, D. Scapillato, S. Miezitis, and B. F. Shaw. (1999). "Cognitive-Behavioral Group Treatments in Childhood Anxiety Disorders: The Role of Parental Involvement." *Journal of the American Academy of Child and Adolescent Psychiatry*, 38 (3): 1223–1229.

Moes, D. (1995). "Parent Education and Parenting Stress." In R. L. Koegel and L. K. Koegel (Eds.), *Teaching Children with Autism: Strategies for*

Initiating Positive Interactions and Improving Learning Opportunities. Baltimore: Paul H Brookes Publishing.

National Research Council. (2001). *Educating Children with Autism.* Washington: National Academy Press.

Osterling, J., G. Dawson, and J. Munson. (2002). "Early Recognition of One-Year-Old Infants with Autism Spectrum Disorder Versus Mental Retardation." *Development and Psychopathology,* 14 (2):239–251.

Patterson, G. R., and G. Brodsky. (1966). "A Behaviour Modification Programme for a Child with Multiple Problem Behaviours." *Journal of Child Psychology and Psychiatry,* 9 (3): 277–295.

Reaven, J., and S. Hepburn. (2003). "Cognitive Behavioral Treatment of Obsessive-Compulsive Disorder in a Child with Asperger Syndrome." *Autism,* 7(3): 145–164.

———. (2006). "The Parent's Role in the Treatment of Anxiety Symptoms in Children with High-Functioning Autism Spectrum Disorders." *Mental Health Aspects of Developmental Disabilities,* 9(1): 73–80.

Robbins, F. R., G. Dunlap, and A. J. Plienis. (1991). "Family Characteristics, Family Training, and the Progress of Young Children with Autism." *Journal of Early Intervention,* 15(2): 173–184.

Rocha, M. L., L. Schreibman, and A. C. Stahmer. (2007). "Effectiveness of Training Parents to Teach Joint Attention in Children with Autism." *Journal of Early Intervention,* 29 (2): 154–172.

Rogers, S. J., and D. DiLalla. (1991). "A Comparative Study of the Effects of a Developmentally Based Instructional Model on Young Children with Autism and Young Children with Other Disorders of Behavior and Development." *Topics in Early Childhood Special Education,* 11(1): 29–48.

Rogers, S. J., and H. Lewis. (1989). "An Effective Day Treatment Model for Young Children with Pervasive Developmental Disorders." *Journal of the American Academy of Child and Adolescent Psychiatry*, 28(2): 207–214.

Rogers, S. J., T. Hall, D. Osaki, J. Reaven, and J. Herbison. (2001). The Denver Model: "A Comprehensive, Integrated, Educational Approach to Young Children with Autism and their Families." In J. S. Handleman and S. L. Harris (Eds.), *Preschool Education Programs for Children with Autism*. Austin, TX: Pro-Ed.

Rogers, S. J., H. C. Lewis, and K. Reis. (1987). "An Effective Procedure for Training Early Special Education Teams to Implement a Model Program." *Journal of the Division of Early Childhood*, 11(2): 180–188.

Rogers, S. J., J. Herbison, H. Lewis, J. Pantone, and K. Reis. (1986). "An Approach for Enhancing the Symbolic, Communicative, and Interpersonal Functioning of Young Children with Autism and Severe Emotional Handicaps." *Journal of the Division of Early Childhood*, 10(2):135–148.

Rogers, S. J., and Ozonoff, S. (2006). Behavioral, Educational, and Developmental Treatments for Autism. In S. O. Moldin and J. L. R. Rubenstein (Eds.), Understanding Autism: From Basic Neuroscience to Treatment. Boca Raton, FL: CRC Press.

Schreibman, L., and R. L. Koegel. (2005). "Training for Parents of Children with Autism: Pivotal Responses, Generalization, and Individualization of Interventions." In E. D. Hibbs and P. S. Jensen (Eds.), *Psychosocial Treatments for Child and Adolescent disorders: Empirically Based Strategies for Clinical Practice*. Washington: American Psychological Association.

Schreibman, L., W. M. Kaneko, and R. L. Koegel. (1991). "Positive Affect of Parents of Autistic Children: A Comparison across two Teaching Techniques." *Behavior Therapy*, 22 (4): 479–490.

Seligman, M. E. P. (1972). "Learned Helplessness." *Annual Review of Medicine,* 23($): 407–412.

Seltzer, M. M., P. Shattuck, L. Abbeduto, and J. S. Greenberg. (2004). "Trajectory of Development in Adolescents and Adults with Autism." *Mental Retardation and Developmental Disabilities Research Reviews*, 10(2):234–247.

Seung, H. K., S. Ashwell, J. H. Elder, and G. Valcante. (2006). "Verbal Communication Outcomes in Children with Autism after In-home Father Training." *Journal of Intellectual Disability Research,* 50 (2): 139–150.

Symon, J. B. (2005). "Expanding Interventions for Children with Autism: Parents as Trainers." *Journal of Positive Behavior Interventions*, 7(2): 159–173.

Sofronoff, K., A. Leslie, and W. Brown. (2004). "Parent Management Training and Asperger Syndrome: A Randomized Controlled Trial to Evaluate a Parent-based Intervention." *Autism*, 8 (3): 301–317.

Stahmer, A. C. (1995). "Teaching Symbolic Play Skills to Children with Autism Using Pivotal Response Training." *Journal of Autism and Developmental Disorders,* 25(2): 123–141.

Stern, J. (2000). "Parent Training." In J. R. White and A. S. Arthur (Eds.), *Cognitive-Behavioral Group Therapy: For Specific Problems and Populations.* Washington: American Psychological Association.

Smith, T., G. A. Buch, and T. E. Gamby. (2000). "Parent-Directed, Intensive Early Intervention for Children with Pervasive Developmental Disorder." *Research in Developmental Disabilities*, 21(3): 297–309.

Smith, T., P. A. Donahoe, and B. J. Davis. (2001). "The UCLA Young Autism Project." In J. S. Handleman and S. L. Harris (Eds.), *Preschool Education Programs for Children with Autism*. Austin, TX: Pro-Ed.

Strain, P. S., and M. Hoyson. (2000). "The Need for Longitudinal Intensive Social Skill Intervention: LEAP Follow-up Outcomes for Children with Autism." *Topics in Early Childhood Special Education*, 20(1): 116–122.

Sze, K. M., and J. J. Wood. (2007). "Cognitive Behavioral Treatment of Comorbid Anxiety Disorders and Social Difficulties in Children with High-Functioning Autism: A Case Report." *Journal of Contemporary Psychotherapy,* 37(2): 133–143.

Volkmar, F., K. Chawarska, and A. Klin. (2005). "Autism in Infancy and Early Childhood". *Annual Review of Psychology,* 56(3): 315–336.

Webster-Stratton, C., and M. J. Reid. (2003). "The Incredible Years Parents, Teachers, and Children Training Series: A Multifaceted Treatment Approach for Young Children with Conduct Problems." In A. E. Kazdin and J. R. Weisz (Eds.), *Evidence-Based Psychotherapies for Children and Adolescents.* New York: Guilford Press.

Weiskop, S., A. Richdale, and J. Matthews. (2005). "Behavioral Treatment to Reduce Sleep Problems in Children with Autism or Fragile X Syndrome." *Developmental Medicine and Child Neurology,* 47(1): 94–104.

Wetherby, A. M., and J. J. Woods. (2006). "Early Social Interaction Project for Children with Autism Spectrum Disorders Beginning in the Second Year of Life: A Preliminary Study." Topics of Early Childhood Special Education, 26 (1): 67–82.

Chapter 15

CONCLUSIONS AND POLICY IMPLICATIONS ON AUTISM SPECTRUM DISORDERS

Introduction

Autism spectrum disorder (ASD) is a neurodevelopmental condition characterized by deficits in social communication and social interactions and restricted, repetitive patterns of behaviors, interests, or activities. ASD is a highly heterogeneous condition with the concept of a spectrum capturing the differences among autistic people in terms of symptoms, intelligence, and language abilities; neuro-psychological underpinnings, which include cognitive style, information processing, and sensory deviations; etiology and comorbidities, as well as the levels of functioning, adaptation, and well-being (American Psychiatric Association, 2013). Autism is a lifelong developmental disability that affects how people perceive, communicate, and interact with others. However, it is essential to recognize that there are different opinions that all autistic people are not disabled. It should be noted that before the Act of Autism, it was often misunderstood by the general people and professionals that autism is a neurological disease, and as a result, most autistic people faced several significant problems to survive at the family, community, and societal levels. To overcome these problems, a plan of action is required to prevent autism, and at the same time, we need to increase the services and support for autistic individuals and their families. It should be communicated that autism is not a disease; instead, it is a developmental disorder due to consanguinity as well as inbreeding. Autism may be prevented by avoiding consanguinity, which is identified as one of its causes. So far, the researcher's knowledge goes that no significant research has been conducted on consanguinity and its effects on autism in Bangladesh. A few studies were conducted in Western countries and some Eastern countries, especially in the Middle East, India, and China, to explore the root causes of autism and how it can be prevented by avoiding consanguineous marriages. Consequently, in many countries, consanguineous marriages have already been discouraged by enacting rules and regulations to reduce autism spectrum disorder (ASD).

Before discussing the policy implications, there is a need to conceptualize how autism is formed and evolves over everyone's lifetime. This will help to determine the ways and timing of policy interventions. Family and twin studies offer strong evidence for a predominant genetic etiology in ASD, with over one hundred susceptibility genes identified to be strongly linked to autism (Wisniowiecka-Kowalnik and Nowakowska 2019) and heritability estimates ranging from 50–95 percent (Lovaas et al. 1973). Although there is a preponderance of genetic factors, the literature suggests that ASD could result from effects derived from environmental risk factors and gene and environment interactions (Berry et al. 2013). However, a deeper understanding of epigenetics has underscored the conceptualization of disorders as a "mismatch between individual and a specific environment, rather than an abnormality per se." It can explain autism as an expected reaction to a non-optimal environment for the individual in a physical and psychosocial context (Hens, 2021). Specifically, in ASD, it is hypothesized that genetic and environmental factors lead to a subject's atypical patterns of interactions with the environment, with impaired engagement in social interactions. These risk processes will result, on the one hand, in abnormal social and linguistic brain circuitry and, eventually, mediate the development of full-blown ASD (i.e., "autism will create itself"). On the other hand, they may intervene through epigenetics in the expression of the susceptibility genes, further strengthening their effects, as if in a vicious cycle (Dawson 2008). Finally, as expected, the overall outcome of autism and its burden is further determined by social, psychological, and biological factors from childhood to adolescence and adulthood through constant feedback loops between the environment and the disorder indices (Levy et al. 2006).

Policies for Bangladesh

Bangladesh has a total population of more than one hundred and seventy million. About 85 percent of the population is Muslim, and consanguineous marriages are allowed and practiced among the Muslim population in different perspectives, viz. quasi-socioeconomic incentives along with political and cultural factors associated with the practice of consanguineous marriages among them. It has been observed that most people do not know the genetic effects of consanguinity in terms of cross-cousin and parallel-cousin marriages upon the offspring or future generations.

The research findings indicate that autism is associated with inbreeding and gene mutation of the offspring whose parents are involved in consanguineous marriages compared to the non-consanguineous marital background of the parents. It is also revealed in different studies that autism may take place among the children of non-consanguineous marriages due to other factors that are discussed elsewhere in this volume. However, their effects are to a lesser extent. Under the circumstances, the results of this research will be able to contribute to the knowledge of the planners, policymakers, practitioners, academics, and researchers along with the general people to take the initiative to prevent consanguinity or consanguineous marriages either cross-cousin or parallel–cousin to get rid of autism which may take place in the inbred community in Bangladesh to improve the quality of life and well being of the future generations which will be helpful for human resource development. Keeping this view, to reduce and prevent autism, the following policies need to be implemented from the grassroots to the national level using the methods and techniques of the participatory approach. It should be mentioned that the policies need to be 'bottom-up' instead of 'top-down' to make the policies sustainable in involving the beneficiaries because the beneficiaries will be stakeholders for the program's continuation in the future.

- **ASD Research and Awareness Platform:** There should be established an ASD research and awareness platform in every district of Bangladesh, which encompasses community-based organizations and a multidisciplinary team including psychiatrists, psychologists, pediatricians, geneticists, public health experts, and social work specialists. Under the platform, autistic people need to be members through registration, and registration facilities need to be created to obtain the basic epidemiological profiles of persons with ASD, epilepsy, and other psychiatric disorders. In addition, through this platform, research should be done on autism to take pragmatic plans of action to prevent it, as well as to provide services to autistic individuals.

- **Avoid Consanguinity by Genetic Counseling:** The study proposes several recommendations to create realistic policies. The most important is to stay away from marrying relatives and initiate awareness programs to show the negative consequences of consanguineous marriages on their offspring through genetic counseling. Genetic counseling is the process by which clients or their relatives at risk of an inherited disorder are advised about the consequences and nature of the disorder, the probabilities of developing or transmitting the genes, and the choices open to them in the management and planning of their families to prevent or avoid or ameliorate the disorder. This has multiple dimensions, such as preventive, diagnostic, therapeutic, and supportive value. Some valuable tips are given in counseling to consanguineous couples.

  ➢ Refer well before conception, especially if they have a family history of a possible autosomal recessive condition.

  ➢ Remember to empathize and not imply that a child's condition is the parents' fault, even if the couple is consanguineous and the child has two identical copies of a mutant gene. Nobody deliberately chooses to pass on an illness to their offspring, and no one is to blame.

  ➢ Ensure that the couple referred for premarital genetic counseling is informed that no blood tests provide 'General Genetic Compatibility' data and that few basic carrier tests are available for a limited range of specific conditions.

> Adopt a nonjudgmental attitude and a positive mindset to disseminate knowledge and information to the couple, empowering them with available options and enabling them to make intelligent decisions.

> Deal with the issue in a sensitive, caring, and sensible manner.

Genetic counseling yields the best results when done premarital or at least prior to conception. A non-judgmental attitude toward consanguineous couples is essential on the part of the counselor to establish good communication channels and to foster effective working relationships between medical professionals and the communities where consanguineous marriages are prevalent (Koegel et al. 1987)

- **Advocacy against Consanguinity:** Genetic counselors act as healthcare team members and patient advocates, protecting their best interests and working as a genetic resource to physicians. Genetic counselors provide helpful information and support to families at risk of an array of inherited disorders. They are involved in identifying families at risk, investigating problems presented by the family, interpreting information about the disorder, analyzing inheritance patterns, and evaluating recurrence risks while reviewing testing options available to the family.

- **Inspiring the Religious Values:** When an abnormality or illness is identified in a child of a consanguineous couple, investigations and referrals must proceed systematically, as clinically indicated for the presenting symptoms, but with an emphasis on autosomal recessive conditions in the diagnosis. Nevertheless, it is essential to remember that autosomal recessive conditions can arise by chance, with the child having two different mutations, not necessarily because of consanguineous marriage alone. This can go a long way in eliminating shame and guilt in the parents, that somehow, they were responsible for the condition of their child, or in erasing the misconception that God is punishing them for their sin of marrying close relatives.

Conclusions and Policy Implications on Autism Spectrum Disorders

- **Consanguineous Couple Need to Be Tested:** A family history of possible autosomal recessive condition may considerably increase offspring risk over consanguinity's background risks. The consanguineous couple can be tested for their carrier status and prenatal diagnosis when necessary. Investigating an affected relative may provide valuable clues when the diagnosis or mutation is unknown. If this is not possible, an estimation of risks involved and detailed, systematic fetal scans are the only choices open. However, this may leave many couples disconcerted by the residual uncertainty.

- **Relevant Genetic Information should be Desiminated:** In the case of death of the affected child or termination of the affected pregnancy, a postmortem examination may throw light on the causal factors. This presents the best chance to diagnose and identify the causal mutation. While being distressful to the grieving parents, this examination may reveal information that may enable their physicians to predict the health status of the next child or children. It is important to remember that it could be highly frustrating for a couple if, in a future pregnancy, the lack of relevant genetic information about their first child makes it impossible to provide accurate advice and testing.

- **Inclusion in Academic Curriculum:** The young age of consanguineous couples further implicates a need to increase awareness programs among the young generation about the deleterious effects of consanguineous marriages through inclusion in the academic curriculum. The social benefits derived from such marriages are paramount to consanguineous couples. However, the availability of preventive measures should be emphasized. Further genetic investigation must be conducted in this area to elucidate the mode of inheritance. Bangladesh must take a giant leap in this direction, where consanguineous marriages are more prevalent. The need of the hour is to set up infrastructure with primary research and good medical facilities for genetic testing and counseling.

- **Introducing the Genetic Testing Facilities:** In many medical college hospitals in Bangladesh, the facilities are meager, and as a result, many spouses do not get a chance to get genetic tests. It has been observed that genetic testing facilities are available with well-trained genetic counselors to handle the situation in a few medical college hospitals, especially at the divisional level. Adopting better translational research concepts and intervention strategies helps consanguineous couples make reproductive decisions they must make throughout their lives.

- **Initiative Should be Taken at the Government Level:** At the governmental level, the relevant governmental agencies should provide and ensure affordability of and accessibility to autism resources, including educational services for autistic children and their caregivers. The various higher education ministries should initiate training programs for teachers to educate them on the appropriate skills needed to give every child with autism the best care. More importantly, there is a desperate need for national policy formulation to care for autistic children in close cooperation with the GOs and NGOs involving the local communities.

- **Intensive Training to the Caregivers:** Intensive training should be given to those directly or indirectly caring for autistic children. The different methods of training the parents of autistic children, viz. naturalistic behavior methods, integrated developmental and behavioral methods, and cognitive behavioral methods, need to be incorporated. At the caregiving level, caregivers should be involved in planning and evaluating autism policies and programs, such as school integration. Similarly, family training and education are essential in passing knowledge and experiences to others through informal contacts. Local associations are critical for promoting parental empowerment and providing formal support services to assist the children and their families in their well-being.

- **Research Foundation Needs to Be Established:** At the research level, a research foundation is needed to integrate research efforts from different countries to standardize screening and diagnostic tools across countries and cultures. Extensive research is also necessary to determine management recommendations and treatment modalities that best suit various cultures across the East and the West for the treatment and rehabilitation of autistic individuals.

- **Holistic Facilities Need to Be Provided:** Holistic facilities mean all sorts of facilities need to be given for the overall development of autistic children. At the organizational level, more centers for treating autism are needed. The current autism centers must increase their capacity to accept more children in their programs and adopt various special educational programs. Special schools are required to have full-fledged facilities to educate autistic children. Vocational rehabilitation for adults with autism is also needed to minimize the costs for families and caregivers. This can be achieved by establishing training colleges and organizations specialized in vocational rehabilitation to raise employers' awareness about the working ability of autistic people. Finally, the public and private sectors must cooperate to ensure that more organized and effective efforts are provided.

- **Peer Training Program and Combination Approach:** A peer training program and combination approach need to be introduced because the studies revealed that autistic children experience intensified feelings of loneliness (Bauminger and Kasari 2000; Chamberlain et al. 2007), possibly reflecting a more nuanced understanding of social integration and relationships over time. In recent years, mapping social networks has shed some light on how students with autism are assimilated and integrated into the larger social environment. Researchers have already examined variables such as the reciprocity of friendship connections. In addition, they have sought more specific information about how to best address the social deficits exhibited with peers, given that the gains of most training approaches are modest (Bellini et al. 2007; Rao et al. 2008; White et al. 2007). In general, approaches that include peers directly in training efforts are much more successful than those that do not include them (Kasari 2008). Both peer training programs and combination approaches are more effective than only teaching the child with autism.

Concluding Remarks

Consanguineous marriages have occurred between people considered relatives and who are usually, but not necessarily, biological kin. Increasingly, in recent years, cousin marriages have come to be regarded as genetically risky. A discourse of genetic risk in marriages between consanguineous kin defined by geneticists as second cousins or closer has been promulgated in public health debate in many countries across the East and the West where cousin marriage is practiced. There has, however, been little systematic comparative analysis to date of how these understandings of genetic risk are being incorporated within state health policies and how they may be influencing traditional forms of spouse selection. This book is an attempt to explore the network relationship of consanguinity, inbreeding, and autism in an inbred community where cross-cousin and parallel-cousin marriages prevailed due to fulfilling the socio-cultural and quasi-economic interest between the bride and groom along with their parents.

References

American Psychiatric Association. (2013). Diagnostic and Statistical Manual of Mental Disorders. Arlington: American Psychiatric Publishing Ltd.

Bauminger, N. and C. Kasari. (2000). "Loneliness and Friendship in High-Functioning Children with Autism." *Child Development,* 71(94): 447–456.

Berry, R. J., K. S. Crider, and M. Yeargin-Allsopp. (2013). "Periconceptional Folic Acid and Risk of Autism Spectrum Disorders." *JAMA,* 309 (4): 611–613.

Bellini, S., J. K. Peters, L. Benner, and A. Hopf. (2007). "A Meta-Analysis of School-Based Social Skills Interventions for Children with Autism Spectrum Disorders." Remedial and Special Education, 28 (2): 153–162.

Chamberlain, B., C. Kasari, and E. Rotheram-Fuller. (2007). "Involvement or Isolation: The Social Networks of Children with Autism in Regular Classrooms." *Journal of Autism and Developmental Disorders,* 37(2): 230–242.

Dawson, G. (2008). "Early Behavioral Intervention, Brain Plasticity and the Prevention of Autism Spectrum Disorder". *Development and Psychopathology,* 20(3): 775–803.

"Epidemiology of Autism Spectrum Disorders." *Annual Review of Public Health,* 38(3): 81–102.

Hens, K. (2021). "The Many Meanings of Autism: Conceptual and Ethical Reflections". *Developmental Medicine and Child Neurology,* 61(3): 1025–1029.

Kasari, C. (2008). "Peer Relationships, Friendships, and Loneliness at School for Children with ASD." Presentation at Organization for Autism Research Annual Research Convocation, Atlanta, GA.

Koegel, R. L., K. Dyer, and L. K. Bell. (1987). "The Influence of Child-Preferred Activities on Autistic Children's Social Behavior." *Journal of Applied Behavior Analysis*, 20 (3): 243–252.

Levy, S., Kim, A., and Olive, M. L. (2006). "Interventions for Young Children with Autism: A Synthesis of the Literature." *Focus on Autism and Other Developmental Disabilities*, 21(1): 55–62.

Lovaas, O. I., R. Koegel, J. Q. Simmons, and J. S. Long. (1973). "Some Generalization and Follow-Up Measures on Autistic Children in Behavior Therapy." *Journal of Applied Behavior Analysis*, 6 (1): 131–166.

Rao, P. A., D. C. Beidel, and M. J. Murray. (2008). "Social Skills Interventions for Children with Asperger's Syndrome or High-Functioning Autism: A Review and Recommendations." *Journal of Autism and Developmental Disorders,* 38(2), 353–361.

White, S. W., K. Keonig, and L. Scahill. (2007). "Social Skills Development in Children with Autism Spectrum Disorders: A Review of the Intervention Research." *Journal of Autism and Developmental Disorders*, 37(10), 1858–1868.

Wisniowiecka-Kowalnik, B., and B. A. Nowakowska. (2019). "Genetics and Epigenetics of Autism Spectrum Disorder-Current Evidence in the Field." *Journal of. Applied. Genetic*, 60 (2):37–47..

Glossary

Asperger Syndrome (AS): A developmental disorder on the autism spectrum. People with AS have average or above-average intelligence and have no significant delay in language development. Many people with AS have challenges with motor planning and motor skills.

Atrial Septal Defect (ASD): An atrial septal defect (ASD) — sometimes called a hole in the heart — is a congenital heart defect in which there is an abnormal opening in the dividing wall between the upper filling chambers of the heart (the atria). In most cases, ASDs are diagnosed and treated successfully with few or no complications.

Atrio-ventricular septal Defect (AVSD): An AVSD occurs when there are holes between the chambers of the right and left sides of the heart. This condition is also called atrioventricular canal (AV canal) defect or endocardial cushion defect. In people with AVSD, the valves that control blood flow between these chambers may not form correctly.

Attention deficit hyperactivity disorder (ADHD): A neurological condition with specific chronic core symptoms, including distractibility, disorganized thinking, poor impulse control, mood shifts, forgetfulness, and hyperactivity. ADHD is believed to affect 3 – 5% of the population.

Atypical autism: A term used in the International Statistical Classification of Diseases and Related Health Problems – Tenth Revision (ICD -10) to describe a condition that differs from autism in terms of either age of onset (an Autistic Disorder diagnosis requires that symptoms are apparent before the age of three) or failure to meet the criteria for Autism in all three areas: reciprocal social interaction, verbal and non-verbal communication, and stereotyped behaviors or restricted interests. In the Diagnostic and Statistical Manual of Mental Disorders – Fourth Edition (DSM IV), it is called Pervasive Developmental Disorder – Not Otherwise Specified (PDD NOS).

Autism: Autism, also known as autism spectrum disorder (ASD), is a neurodevelopmental disorder that affects brain development. There is no one type of autism or how it appears in children.

Autism Spectrum Disorder (ASD): Autism is often referred to as a "spectrum disorder," meaning that the symptoms and characteristics of autism can present themselves in a variety of combinations, ranging from mild to severe. The Autistic Spectrum includes Autistic Disorder (AD), Asperger Syndrome (AS), and Pervasive Developmental Disorder – Not Otherwise Specified (PDD-NOS). Childhood Disintegrative Disorder and Retts Disorder are not usually considered part of the Autistic Spectrum. However, they are grouped with them in the Diagnostic and Statistical Manual of the American Psychiatric Association (DSM-IV).

Autistic Disorder: "(Also called autism.) a neurological and developmental disorder that usually appears during the first three years of life. A child with autism appears to live in their world, showing little interest in others and a lack of social awareness. The focus of an autistic child is a consistent routine and includes an interest in repeating odd and peculiar behaviors. Autistic children often have problems in communication, avoid eye contact, and show limited attachment to others."

Bio-social institution: "Biosocial" is a broad concept referencing the dynamic, bidirectional interactions between biological phenomena and social relationships and contexts, constituting human development processes over the life course.

Bipolar disorders: Bipolar disorder (formerly called manic-depressive illness or manic depression) is a mental illness that causes unusual shifts in a person's mood, energy, activity levels, and concentration. These shifts can make it difficult to carry out day-to-day tasks.

Case Study: A case study is a research methodology in social and life sciences. There is no one definition of case study research.[1] However, very simply... a case study can be defined as an intensive study about a person, a group of people, or a unit, which is aimed to generalize over several units.

Central Coherence: Individuals with autism spectrum disorders are said to have "weak central coherence," which is the capacity to integrate information to make sense of one's environment. People with autism tend to focus on details and process information piecemeal rather than on a situation's context and overall meaning (They have trouble understanding the gist, the "whole picture," or the gestalt).

Central Coherence: Central coherence is a concept that describes the ability to derive meaning from a mass of details. Someone with strong central coherence looking at a forest will see the trees but recognize they make up a bigger concept -- a forest.

Cerebral Cortex: The outer layer of the brain's gray matter is where higher brain functions, such as sensation, voluntary movement, thought, reasoning, and memory.

Child Neglect: Child neglect is defined as any egregious act or omission by a parent or other caregiver that deprives a child of basic age-appropriate needs and thereby results or has a reasonable potential to result, in physical or psychological harm.

Childhood Autism Rating Scale (CARS): A brief rating scale measures the severity of autism in a child over two years of age based on ratings of fifteen individual behavioral characteristics. The total score may fall in the "non-autistic," "autistic," or "severely autistic" ranges. It is usually based on the professional's observations of the child's behavior, although some information may be obtained by interviewing a parent or caregiver. Special training is required to use the CARS.

Childhood Disintegrative Disorder: A relatively rare condition that resembles autism occurring in 3- and 4-year-olds, characterized by a deterioration of intellectual, social, and language functioning from previously normal functioning. A Pervasive Developmental Disorder, although not included as an autism spectrum disorder.

Childhood-onset Pervasive Developmental Disorders: Pervasive developmental disorders (PDD) — now known as autism spectrum disorder — are a group of developmental delays that affect social and communication skills. The typical onset of PDD occurs around age 3, but some parents notice symptoms during infancy. Treatment typically involves therapy and medications.

Chromosome: A structure (typically 46 in humans) in the cell nucleus is the genes' bearer.

Co-existing Disorders: In addition to cognitive impairments, individuals with ASD often suffer from multiple psychopathologies. These include impulse-control disorders, psychoses, obsessive-compulsive disorder, seizures, mood and anxiety disorders, and developmental delays. They are also called co-morbid disorders, differential diagnoses, or dual diagnoses.

Cognitive Behavioral Therapy: Cognitive behavioral therapy (CBT) is a form of psychological treatment that has been demonstrated to be effective for a range of problems, including depression, anxiety disorders, alcohol and drug use problems, marital problems, eating disorders, and severe mental illness.

Cognitive Behavioral Therapy: A treatment that combines behavior therapy with cognitive therapy and that works to reduce habitual reactions to challenging situations. CBT assists the person in learning how specific ways of thinking may cause or contribute to feelings of anxiousness, depression, or anger that, in turn, lead to negative behavior.

Communication Disorder: Any interference with a person's ability to comprehend or express ideas, experiences, knowledge, or feelings.

Co-morbidity: When a person has two or more different conditions simultaneously, these conditions are said to be co-morbid. For example, a person can have both Fragile X syndrome and Autism or an anxiety disorder and Autism. (See also: Co-existing Disorders).

Comprehensive Diagnostic Evaluation: A comprehensive diagnostic evaluation for autism is a meticulous and thorough assessment process. Professionals conduct it to determine the presence of autism spectrum disorder. A comprehensive diagnostic evaluation for autism aims to gather comprehensive information, including the individual's developmental history and behavioral patterns.

Congenital: A condition that is present from birth.

Consanguineous Marriage: Consanguineous marriage is a marriage between closely related individuals.

Consanguinity: Consanguinity is usually defined as the result of a sexual reproduction between two related individuals. It can also refer to populations sharing at least one common ancestor, such as those who live within isolated communities or practice endogamy.

Cranio-sacral Therapy (CST): Using a soft touch, therapists relieve blockages in the craniosacral system, the membranes, and cerebrospinal fluid surrounding the brain and spinal cord to improve the functioning of the central nervous system. This therapy is controversial.

Cousin marriage: Cousin marriage, or consanguineous marriage, involves two people related as cousins, typically second cousins or more closely related, getting married and starting a family together. Cousin marriage has been prevalent throughout history and is still practiced in many societies worldwide.

Data Analysis: Data Analysis systematically applies statistical and/or logical techniques to describe, illustrate, condense, recap, and evaluate data.

Data Editing: Data editing is the application of checks to detect missing, invalid or inconsistent entries or to point to data records that are potentially in error.

Data Processing: Data processing refers to essential operations executed on raw data to transform the information into a useful format or structure that provides valuable insights to a user or organization. The outcomes of data processing operations flow into various data outputs as designed by a data scientist, including data analytics, business intelligence, machine learning (ML) and artificial intelligence (AI).

Delayed Milestones: Milestones are the predicted points when a child reaches a significant stage in development, such as walking or talking. A delayed milestone occurs when a child has not reached a significant stage at the predicted age.

Demographic profile: A demographic profile combines social and demographic factors defining people in a specific group or population.

Detrimental effects: Detrimental effects by the use due to its nature, include noise that exceeds sound levels normally found in residential areas, environmental impacts, dust, fumes, smoke, odor, noise, vibrations; chemicals, toxins, pathogens, gases, heat, light, electromagnetic disturbances, and radiation.

Developmental Disability: It is defined as "measured intellectual functioning of approximately 70 IQ or lower, with onset before age 18, and measured significant limitations in two or more adaptive skill areas."

Developmental Language Disorder: Children have language disorders when they have problems expressing their thoughts, understanding written material, or what others say. The disorder is developmental when it presents itself as the child grows and does not result from injury.

Developmental Level: A method of observing how children achieve developmental milestones, particularly those related to a child's ability to stay engaged, express mutual pleasure and attention, engage in complex problem-solving and symbolic play, and link ideas

Developmental Screening: Developmental screening involves partnerships with parents to identify child development concerns.

Developmental, Individual-Difference, Relationship-Based (DIR): Developmental, Individual-Difference, Relationship-Based (DIR), also known as DIR/Floortime, is a framework that helps clinicians, parents, and educators conduct a comprehensive assessment and develop an intervention program tailored to the unique challenges and strengths of children with autism spectrum disorders (ASD) and other developmental challenges. The objectives of the DIR®/Floor time™ Model are to build healthy foundations for social, emotional, and intellectual capacities.

Developmentally Delayed (DD): An informal term describes the development of children who cannot perform the skills that other children of the same age can usually perform or who accomplish developmental "milestones" (sitting, walking, first words, etc.) at a significantly slower pace than average. A preferred term by many instead of the medical term 'mental retardation.'

Diagnosis Features of ASD: Numerous diagnostic guidelines of varying quality are available. The essential features of ASD diagnosis include observing a child's relationship and exchange with their parents and an individual unknown to the child during unstructured and structured assessment activities and a detailed history of the child's development.

Diagnostic and Statistical Manual of Mental Disorders (DSM-III): The Diagnostic and Statistical Manual of Mental Disorders, Third Edition (DSM-III), published by the American Psychiatric Association in 1980 and now translated into many languages, has raised great interest worldwide. The evolution of psychiatric nosology and the circumstances of the birth of DSM-III are described.

Disorder's heterogeneity: A term that describes when different gene mutations (changes) cause the same disease or condition.

Down Syndrome: Down syndrome is a naturally occurring chromosomal arrangement that has always been a part of the human condition. The occurrence of Down syndrome is universal across racial and gender lines, and it is present in approximately one in 800 births in Canada.

DSM-IV Diagnostic and Statistical Manual of Mental Disorders: Mental health professionals thus use the DSM-IV codes to describe the features of a given mental disorder and indicate how the disorder can be distinguished from other similar problems. The coding system utilized by the DSM-IV is designed to correspond with codes from the International Classification of Diseases, Ninth Revision, and Clinical Modification, commonly referred to as the ICD-9-CM.

Echolalia: She is repeating words or phrases heard previously. The echoing may occur immediately after hearing the word or phrase or much later. Delayed echolalia can occur days or weeks after hearing the word or phrase. (Canadian Autism Intervention Network)

Emotional Abuse: Emotional abuse includes non-physical behaviors that are meant to control, isolate, or frighten you. This may present in romantic relationships as threats, insults, constant monitoring, excessive jealousy, manipulation, humiliation, intimidation, and dismissiveness.

Epilepsy: Epilepsy is not a disease or a psychological disorder but rather a seizure disorder caused by sudden bursts of electrical energy in the brain.

Evidence of Autism Spectrum Disorders: The available facts or information indicate whether a belief or proposition is valid for autism spectrum disorders.

Executive Control: The ability to carry out goal-directed behavior using complex mental processes and cognitive abilities.

Felt Unpleasant Emotion: Negative emotions are unpleasant and disruptive emotional reactions. Examples of negative emotions include sadness, fear, anger, or jealousy. These feelings aren't just unpleasant; they also make it hard to function in your normal daily life, and they interfere with your ability to accomplish goals.

Fragile X Syndrome: The most common cause of inherited mental retardation, with an incidence of about 1/1500 in males and 1/2500 in females. The inheritance pattern of the disease is unlike other X-linked disorders because it shows significant numbers of apparently unaffected male carriers and some clinically affected females. The disease derives its name from a fragile site on the X chromosome of affected individuals.

Gene: Originally defined as the physical unit of heredity, genes are best defined as the unit of inheritance that occupies a specific locus on a chromosome, the existence of which can be confirmed by the occurrence of different allelic forms. Genes are formed from DNA, carried on the chromosomes, and responsible for the inherited characteristics that distinguish one individual from another. Each human individual has an estimated 100,000 separate genes.

Gene Mutation through Consanguinity: Consanguineous marriages are known to result in offspring carrying homozygous mutations. Many autosomal-recessive gene mutations can increase due to consanguineous unions.

Genetic Counselling: Genetic counseling is available to individuals, families, or couples. It is a way to learn about genetic or hereditary disorders and the chance they are passed on to future generations. This information helps people decide about their health, pregnancies, and children's health.

Genotypes: A genotype is a scoring of the type of variant present at a given location (i.e., a locus) in the genome. It can be represented by symbols. For example, BB, Bb, bb could be used to represent a given variant in a gene.

High Functioning Autism (HFA): Individuals with autism who are not cognitively impaired are called 'high functioning.'

Impact of Consanguinity: Parental consanguinity is a predisposing factor for many multifactorial complications, including obesity, cardiovascular disorders, diabetes, and some malignancies, which may influence reproductive outcomes.

Inbreeding: Inbreeding and consanguinity are interchangeable to describe unions between couples with at least one common ancestor. Inbreeding in population genetic terms refers to a departure from non-random "mating" in which individuals' "mate" with those more similar (genetically) to them than if they "mated at random" in the population.

Infant morbidity: Number of infant deaths per 1,000 live births in a calendar year, where an infant is defined as being less than 365 days old.

Infantile autism: Infantile autism is a developmental disability characterized by the onset of disturbances in social and language development before the age of 30 months. It must be distinguished from several disorders, including mental retardation and schizophrenia.

Integrated Behavioral Methods: A function of attitudes toward behavior and perceived norms and personal agency toward that behavior is the most important predictor that a desired behavior will occur.

Kinship ties: Kinship is the most universal and basic of all human relationships. It is based on ties of blood, marriage, or adoption. There are two basic kinds of kinship ties: those based on blood that trace descent and those based on marriage, adoption, or other connections.

Mental Retardation: This medical term refers to significantly below-average intelligence (IQ of 70 or less) that manifests during the developmental period and coexists with adaptive behavior impairments.

Mild Autism Disorder: Mild autism is diagnosed as a level 1 autism spectrum disorder. It means a person does not have intense autism traits and needs a lower level of support than other autistic people often do.

Miscarriages: Miscarriage is the sudden loss of a pregnancy before the 20th week. About 10% to 20% of known pregnancies end in miscarriage.

Mortality: The number of deaths in a population during a given time or place: the proportion of deaths to population.

Natural Language Paradigm (NDP): NLP is also the acronym for something else: "Neuro-Linguistic Programming," and partly for this reason, "Natural Language Paradigm" has been renamed "Pivotal Response Training." See Pivotal Response Training

Naturalistic Behavioral Methods: Naturalistic Developmental Behavioral Intervention (NDBI) is a research-based system for increasing the skills of children who have delays in speech-language communication.

Neonatal: A newborn infant, or neonate, is a child under 28 days of age. During these first 28 days of life, the child is at highest risk of dying. Most newborn deaths take place in developing countries where access to health care is low.

Neurotypical: The word "neurotypical" refers to people who have brains that function similarly to most of their peers. Neurotypical individuals develop skills, such as social or organizational skills, at around the same rate as others their age.

Nonverbal Communication: Nonverbal communication means conveying information without using words.

American Psychological Association: This might involve using certain facial expressions or hand gestures to make a specific point, or it could involve using (or non-use) eye contact, physical proximity, and other nonverbal cues to get a message across.

Observation Method: Observational methods are research techniques used to systematically collect data by observing and documenting behaviors, events, or phenomena as they naturally occur in real-world settings.

Obsessive-Compulsive Disorder (OCD): Obsessions are thoughts or images that are involuntary, intrusive, and anxiety-provoking. Compulsions are impulses to perform a variety of stereotyped behaviors or rituals. OCD is a neurological disorder that causes uncertainty. In OCD, obsessive thoughts and compulsive actions interfere significantly with the individual's daily life, causing marked anxiety and stress.

Parallel cousin marriage: Parallel cousin marriage is marriage between the children of same-sex siblings. Say a mother's daughter marries her sister's son. These two newlyweds would result from parallel cousin marriage, where the children of two sisters or brothers marry.

Parental Stress: Parental stress is a distinct type of stress that arises when a parent's perception of the demands of parenting outstrips his or her resources.

Pervasive Developmental Disorder (PDD): An 'umbrella term' for a group of developmental disorders, which includes Autistic Disorder, Asperger Disorder, Rett Syndrome, and Childhood Disintegrative Disorder. It also consists of a "residual category" of Pervasive Developmental Disorder – Not Otherwise Specified.

Pervasive Developmental Disorder-Not Otherwise Specified (PDD-NOS): Pervasive developmental disorder not otherwise specified (PDD-NOS) falls under the diagnostic category of pervasive developmental disorders (PDD), a group of disorders that is characterized by delays in the development of different basic functions, including communication and socialization.

Pulmonary Atresia (PA): Pulmonary atresia (PA) is a heart defect. It happens when the baby's heart doesn't form as it should in the uterus. This can happen during the first 8 weeks of pregnancy.

Pulmonary Stenosis (PS): Pulmonary valve stenosis is a type of heart valve disease that involves narrowing the pulmonary valve, which controls blood flow from the heart's right ventricle into the pulmonary artery to carry blood to the lungs.

Regression of Milestones: Developmental regression is an expected and self-protective response to hospitalization across all age groups. It is a healthy way for many children to cope with the hospital experience and typically resolves when daily patterns and activities return to normal. An age-related approach to the behavioral changes associated with hospitalization highlights the development continuum.

Rehabilitation Strategies: The rehabilitation strategy aims to reduce the burden of disease and improve functioning as defined in the International Classification of Functioning, Disability, and Health.

Residual autism: Residual autism: individuals who had a history of having autistic disorder but presently do not meet the criteria for autistic disorder (i.e., still having some autistic features after effective interventions and/or natural development)

Self-stimulatory Behaviors: Self-stimulatory behavior is repetitive, stereotyped, functionally autonomous behavior seen in both normal and developmentally disabled populations. Yet, no satisfactory theory of its development and major characteristics has previously been offered.

Sensory Sensitivities: Sensory processing sensitivity (SPS), or environmental sensitivity (ES), is a biologically based trait characterized by increased environmental awareness and sensitivity. A highly sensitive person — whether a child or adult — processes sensory stimuli and information more strongly and deeply than others.

Sexual Abuse: Child sexual abuse is any interaction between a child and an adult (or another child) in which the child is used for the sexual stimulation of the perpetrator or an observer. Sexual abuse can include both touching and non-touching behaviors.

Signs of Social Awkwardness: Social awkwardness may also be confused with the personality trait of introversion. First described by psychoanalyst Carl Jung, introversion and extraversion are opposing psychological preferences that describe how individuals focus and gather their energy. While extroverts look to the outer world, introverts orient themselves inward.

Social demography: Social demography deals with questions of population composition and change and how they interact with sociological variables at the individual and contextual levels.

Social Isolation: Social isolation is the need for more social contacts and having few people to interact with regularly. You can live alone and not feel lonely or socially isolated, and you can feel lonely while being with others.

Stereotyped behaviors: Behaviors in an individual (with autism, for example) that are repeated many times.

Stigmatization: Stigmatization involves identifying and marking an undesirable characteristic in a way that narrows a person's social identity to that characteristic. The consequences of stigmatization include marginalization and, in some cases, dehumanization.

Stillbirths: Stillbirth is when a baby dies in the womb after 20 weeks of pregnancy. Most stillbirths happen before a pregnant person goes into labor, but a small number happen during labor and birth.

Stimming: Stimming is repetitive movements or noises. Stimming seems to help some autistic children and teenagers manage emotions and cope with overwhelming situations.

Survey Method: A survey method is a process, tool, or technique that you can use to gather information in research by asking questions to a predefined group of people. Typically, it facilitates the exchange of information between the research participants and the person or organization carrying out the research.

Symbols of Kinship Relations: They use standardized symbols to represent different types of relationships. For example, a circle typically represents a female and a triangle represents a male.

Temper Tantrums: Temper tantrums range from whining and crying to screaming, kicking, hitting, and breath-holding spells. They're equally common in boys and girls and usually happen between the ages of 1 to 3.

Theory of Mind: Theory of Mind is the branch of cognitive science that investigates how we ascribe mental states to other persons and how we use the states to explain and predict the actions of those other persons.

Ventricular Septal Defect (VSD): A ventricular septal defect (VSD) is a hole in the heart that's present at birth (congenital heart defect). The hole is between the lower heart chambers (right and left ventricles). It allows oxygen-rich blood to move back into the lungs instead of being pumped to the rest of the body.

Verbal Communication: Verbal communication is the most obvious and understood mode of communication, and it is certainly a powerful tool in your communication toolbox. Put, verbal communication is the sharing of information between two individuals using words.

Index

A

abnormal eating behavior, 65
academic learning, 166
acquired gene mutation (SGM), 75
age, 50
age structure, 25, 49, 51, 56
anxiety, 137
Aryan Hindus, 14
Asperger syndrome, 24, 57, 207–9, 212, 214, 227–28
Assisted Reproductive Technology (ART), 160–61
attention deficit hyperactivity disorder (ADHD), 100, 227
autism, etiology of, 68, 82–83, 96
autism spectrum disorder (ASD), xiii–xv, 8–11, 15, 20–26, 60–62, 65–71, 73–74, 81–83, 95–97, 99–101, 108–17, 126–34, 145–53, 155–56, 159–61, 163–66, 171–85, 194, 202–19, 222–26
   causes of, 65
   challenges for parents families, 117–26
   characteristics, 66–67
   diagnostic features of, 103
   diagnostic guideline, 104, 233
   diagnostic tools of, 103
   health management, 107
   myths about, 84–95
   signs and symptoms of, 100–101
   treatment processes of, 105–7
autistic children
   challenges to, 137–42
   family types of, 53–54
autosomal recessive condition, 23, 187–88, 219–21

B

Bangladesh, xv–xvi, 5, 8, 15, 40–42, 59–61, 77–78, 109, 131, 134, 145–53, 155, 182–87, 190, 217–18, 221–22, 247
behavioral intervention, 196, 199–200, 237
   naturalistic, 201
behaviors, self-stimulatory, 118, 133
Breastfeeding, 164
Buddhism, 2, 5–7, 14, 18, 39–41

C

caregivers, 104, 117, 120, 123–24, 196, 222–23, 229
Case Study Method, 29
Center for Neurodevelopment and Autism in Children (CNAC), 145
child neglect, 136
Christianity, 2, 5–6, 14, 41
comorbidities vigilance, 170
comprehensive diagnostic evaluation, 102
congenital hypothyroidism, 161, 187
consanguineous couples, 188
consanguineous marriage, 190
consanguineous marriages, xiii–xiv, 2, 7–15, 18, 25–26, 34–38, 40–45, 56, 61, 67, 69–70, 72–73, 77–80, 146, 160, 182–84, 186–87, 190, 192, 217–21
consanguinity, xiii–xv, 8–12, 14–15, 17–23, 31, 35–36, 38–39, 41–42, 45–48, 69, 71–72, 75, 77–80, 155, 182, 184, 188, 190, 192–93, 217–18
   in Buddhism, 39
   in Christianity, 39
   in Hinduism, 38
   in Islam, 36
cousin marriages, 7–8, 13, 15, 20–23, 26, 37, 45, 67, 70–71, 74, 77, 224, 231
   parallel, 26, 28, 42–43, 46, 72
   patrilineal, 9
cross-cousin marriages, 14, 26, 42–43, 72
   patrilateral, 42, 72

cues, social-emotional, 63, 66, 90, 108, 132

D

data analysis, 30, 231–32
data collection, xvi, 28–29
data editing, xvi, 30, 232
data processing, 30
delayed milestones, 62–63, 232
de novo mutations, 76
developmental screening, 101–2, 233
Developmental Social Pragmatic (DSP), 202
Dhaka City, 27
Disability Rights Law, 147–48, 150
Discrete Trial Training (DTT), 195
disruptive behavior development (DBD), 194
DNA sequence, 74

E

early intervention, 85, 100, 105, 112, 121, 212
Early Start Denver Model (ESDM), 202
eating behavior, abnormal, 65
education, 51
emotional abuse, 9, 135–36, 234
epigenetics, 156–57, 217, 226
Ethical Issues, 161

F

family authority, 54
family cognitive-behavioral therapy (FCBT), 203

first-cousin marriages, 8, 12–13, 37, 40–41
focus group discussion (FGD), 28–29

G

gene mutation, 9, 25–26, 44, 70–71, 73–75, 77, 79, 160, 184, 218, 234–35
genetic changes, 65, 76
genetic counseling, 183–85, 189, 219–20
genetic counselor, 187–88, 220
genetic disorders, 40, 65, 73, 76–78, 92, 155, 182, 184–85
genetics, Mendelian theory of, 44, 73
gestational diabetes, 162

H

Hallervorden-Spatz syndrome (HSS), 9, 17, 191
Hereditary Gene Mutation (HGM), 75
high-functioning autism (HFA), 24, 102, 108–9, 169, 215, 226
Hinduism, 2–5, 8–9, 14, 38, 40
human life, 157–58

I

immune reactions, 163
inbreeding, xiv–xv, 8–9, 14, 19–20, 22–23, 25–26, 31, 34–35, 48, 73–74, 79–80, 146, 155, 160, 184, 192–93, 217–18, 224
inbreeding depression, 73, 79–80
inclusion, 221

inherited inborn disorders, 185
interpregnancy intervals, 163
intracytoplasmic sperm injection, 161
Islam, 2, 4, 13, 23, 40

K

key informants (KI), xv, 28–29

L

language communication, 133

M

marriage, 1–7, 9–13, 15, 17–19, 23, 34–42, 48, 54, 59, 70, 72, 121–22, 130, 158, 160, 182, 188, 192, 221, 224
maternal folic acid supplementation, 164
maternal influenza, 163
maternal obesity, 162
maternal smoking, 162
matriarchal authority structure, 55
matrilateral cross-cousin marriages, 42–44, 72–73
milestones, regression of, 65, 239
Ministry of Health and Family Welfare (MoHFW), 147
Muhammad, Prophet Hazrat, 37
Muslims, 3–5, 11, 13, 17, 19, 40–42, 182, 190, 218
mutations, somatic, 74–76

N

National Autism Academy, 146
National Autism Day, 151
National Plan of Action, 152

Neurodevelopmental Disability Protection Trust Act, 147–48, 150
Newborn Screening (NBS), 114, 185–87, 191
nonverbal communication, 62, 64, 108, 123, 139, 203, 237
North India, 8, 14, 39
nutrient deficiencies, 164

O

observation methods, 28–29
One Stop Mobile Service, 146
Orthodox Church, 15, 41

P

parallel-cousin marriages, xiv, 12–14, 25–26, 44, 72, 146, 218, 224
parental engagement, 166
parental involvement, 204, 211
parental psychopathology, 205
Parental Stress, 117–18, 205, 209, 238
parent-child interactions, 197
parent training intervention, 194, 196–99, 202, 204, 206–7, 209–10, 212, 214
patriarchal authority structure, 54–55
pervasive developmental disorders (PDDs), 61, 93, 100–101, 155, 177, 212, 214. See also autism spectrum disorder (ASD)
physical abuse, 134–35
pollutions, 161
Positive Parenting Program (PPP), 194
practice assignments, home-based, 197–98
premarital counseling, 185
premature birth, 162
prenatal screening, 186
prevention strategies, 156, 158–60, 167, 169, 173
Putra, 4

R

recessive conditions, 44, 71, 73
red flags, 64
regulations, 133
rehabilitation, 164
research design, 22, 27
research report, xv–xvi, 30–31
Roman Catholic Church, 2, 15, 39, 41

S

screening tools, 105
sex, 3–4, 47, 54, 79
sexual abuse, 136
Sheikh Hasina, 148–49
social awkwardness, 63, 240
social demography, 49, 240
social skills, 170
socio-demographic profile, 49
South Asian Autism Network (SAAN), 149
South India, 9, 17, 38, 191
stimming, 65, 137, 240
structure, occupational, 52
survey method, 29, 240

T

temper tantrums, 65, 241

U

United Nations General Assembly, 146, 150

V

verbal communication, 64, 104, 123, 137, 200, 241
vocalizations, spontaneous, 197
vocational rehabilitation, 97, 223

W

Wazed, Saima, 150–51
World Autism Awareness Day, 147, 152
   eleventh, 151

About the Authors

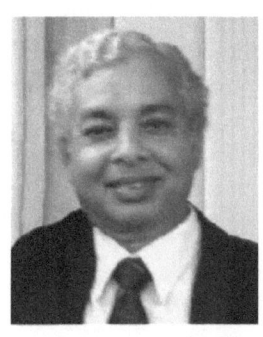

Dr. Profulla C. Sarker did his BA (Hon's) and MA in Social Work in 1971 and 1973, respectively, from the Department of Social Work, University of Rajshahi. He obtained an MPhil. In Sociology 1978 from the Institute of Bangladesh Studies of the same University. He did a PhD in Anthropology from the Department of Anthropology, Centre for Advanced Study, University of Ranchi, India, in 1986. Professor P. C. Sarker is the author of twenty books and co-authored three books published in Dhaka, New Delhi, Singapore, and Toronto University Press. To his credit, he has more than one hundred scientific research papers published in different national and international journals. He is the editor of three journals and a member of the Editorial Board of six international journals. He has supervised eighteen PhD and five MPhil. Dissertations.

Dr. Profulla C. Sarker is the vice chancellor of Sheikh Hasina University of Science and Technology and Adviser to the Royal University of Dhaka. Dr. Sarker was the former pro-vice chancellor of the European University of Bangladesh and the vice chancellor of Prime University, Dhaka. He was a professor and former chairman of the Department of Social Work at the University of Rajshahi, Bangladesh. Dr. Sarker was a professor of Social Work and Social Administration, chairman of the Teachers' Students' Relation Committee, former director of the Institute for Cross-Cultural Studies, and dean of the Division of Social Science and Humanities of Hong Kong Baptist University-Beijing Normal University, UIC, China.

Moreover, he was a senior policy advisor for the National Food Security and Surveillance Project of the Bangladesh Government and the European Commission.

Professor Sarker served as a member of the Curriculum Board of the Regional Center for Social Development, Latrobe University, Australia. He was one of the organizers of the Fourteenth International Congress of Anthropological and Ethnological Sciences held in Virginia, USA, in 1998. Professor P. C. Sarker was a member of the International Scientific Committee of the International Seminars on Health. Mental Health and Social Work was held in Melbourne in 1999 and Tempare, Finland, in 2001. He was a member of the International Scientific Committee of the Third International Conference on Anthropology and the History of Health and Diseases held in Genova, Italy, 2002. He received the Award on Social Development from the International Consortium for Social Development (ICSD), Australia, and the Sir Jagodish Chandra Basu Award on Education and Research in 2018.

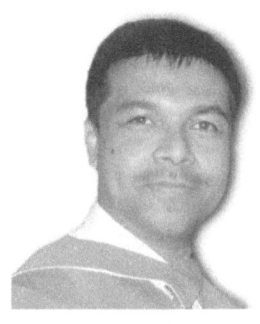
Dr. Nazir M Hossain is a trained clinician who obtained his MBBS from Rajshahi Medical College, Bangladesh, in 1997. Dr. Hossain traveled to the United States of America for his higher study in public health and secured a MPH degree with an Outstanding Scholastic Achievement Award at the Florida International University, USA, in 2001. During his MPH study, he extensively researched "Global Infant Mortality Reasons and Solution" and worked with several government-funded projects on health promotion. To learn more about research on public health and its specialized units, in the year 2004, Dr. Hossain started his Master's in Epidemiology and Biostatistics at Western University of Canada. (Previously, it was Western Ontario University), in which he had done community-based research on Prescription and Non-prescription Medication Use in Pregnancy. In 2005, he was awarded the most prestigious scholarship from York University of Canada to pursue his Doctoral degree in Epidemiology. Dr. Nazir M Hossain completed his PhD in 2011 with a thesis on "Immigrant Children's Health in Canada." Dr. Hossain obtained education and experience in Health Services and Policy Research from the Ontario Training Centre under The Ontario Provincial Ministry of Health and Long-term Care. During his tenure as a researcher with various institutes, he has authored several articles and published them in industry-famous journals. He also co-authored a few government publications. Dr. Hossain has presented several research works at national and international conferences and delivered speeches in many institutes in the last two decades.

Dr. Hossain's expertise and relevance in the field of public health were demonstrated when he became one of the crucial members of the 2009 "Swine Flu Pandemic Preparatory Task Force of Canada." This role showcased his ability to contribute to critical health initiatives and his dedication to public health research. Dr. Nazir M Hossain was also one of the researchers for the historical scenario-building project, "Evidence-based Visions of the Future," with the Public Health Agency of Canada (PHAC) under the Ministry of Health, Canada. To extend his research in public health during disaster situations, he started working with Canada's leading Disaster and emergency management Professionals. Later, He obtained a Master in Disaster and Emergency Management degree from York University.

Dr. Hossain is an adjunct faculty member in the Department of Global Health at York University, Canada. He is also affiliated with Wilfred Laurier University, Canada, and has academic relations with several other post-secondary institutes in Canada. In addition, he has also been working as a consultant to the private and public sectors for the last decade. He is the reviewer for almost a dozen prestigious academic journals.

Dr. Nazir M Hossain and Dr. Profulla C. Sarker have a rich history of collaborative research, with their current project holding significant potential. Their initial work on Arsenic and its impact on reproductive health was presented in Australia in 2001. Now, their research on Inbreeding and Autism from the perspective of Bangladesh has the potential to make a substantial contribution to the field, a prospect that is eagerly anticipated by the academic and professional community.

www.ingramcontent.com/pod-product-compliance
Lightning Source LLC
Chambersburg PA
CBHW020634220526
45464CB00001B/139